Sociology, Health and the Fractured Society

It is now accepted that many of the determinants of health and health care are social. This volume offers a philosophical and theoretical frame within which the nature and extent of this might be optimally examined. The analysis is rooted in Roy Bhaskar's *basic* and *dialectical* critical realism, although it draws also on the critical theory of Jurgen Habermas. It purports to provide an ontologically and epistemologically grounded comparative sociology of contemporary health and health care in the twenty-first century.

Carrying a fourfold agenda, the volume sets out a dialectical critical realist frame for a sociology of health and health care; it clarifies sociology's potential and limitations; it suggests a research programme and a series of questions for investigation; and it offers an argument for an action sociology embedded in a dialectical theory of transformative action.

This volume will be of interest to students and scholars in the areas of philosophy, sociology and critical realism, as well as those working in health and social care.

Graham Scambler was Professor of Medical Sociology at UCL until his retirement in 2013 and is currently Emeritus Professor of Sociology at UCL and Visiting Professor of Sociology at Surrey University.

Routledge Studies in Critical Realism

For a full list of titles in this series, please visit www.routledge.com

Sociology, Health and the Fractured Society

A Critical Realist Account

Graham Scambler

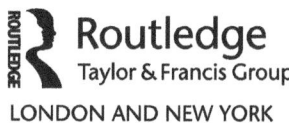

Routledge
Taylor & Francis Group

LONDON AND NEW YORK

First published 2018 by Routledge

2 Park Square, Milton Park, Abingdon, Oxfordshire OX14 4RN

52 Vanderbilt Avenue, New York, NY 10017

Routledge is an imprint of the Taylor & Francis Group, an informa business

First issued in paperback 2019

British Library Cataloguing-in-Publication Data
A catalogue record for this book is available from the British
Library

Library of Congress Cataloging-in-Publication Data
Names: Scambler, Graham, author.
Title: Sociology, health and the fractured society: a critical
realist account / Graham Scambler.
Description: Milton Park, Abingdon, Oxon; New York, NY:
Routledge, 2018. |
Series: Routledge studies in critical realism | Includes
bibliographical references and index.
Identifiers: LCCN 2017053108
Subjects: LCSH: Health—Social aspects. | Social medicine. |
Medicine—Philosophy.
Classification: LCC RA418 .S296 2018 | DDC 362.1—dc23
LC record available at https://lccn.loc.gov/2017053108

ISBN: 978-1-138-90982-3 (hbk)
ISBN: 978-0-367-27173-2 (pbk)

Typeset in Times New Roman
by codeMantra

Contents

Acknowledgements

Much is owed, as ever, to predecessors and consociates. This is a work of 'meta-reflection' indebted equally to social and critical theorists and to empirical researchers.

More than this, I pay tribute to the late Roy Bhaskar's pioneering and creative philosophical underlabouring and to his generosity of spirit. Like many, I miss conversing with him. He didn't just talk philosophy and sociology: whenever we met he asked after Annette and our four daughters. I still owe much to the remarkable work of Jurgen Habermas, as will be apparent. Finally, Margaret Archer too has been a source of inspiration as well as always being a pleasure to meet and debate with. There are occasions in which I question my 'only child' predilection for secreting myself away to write alone! But then …

The book is dedicated to Annette Scambler, sociologist and feminist, who puts up with a lot with remarkable forbearance.

Introduction

My orientation to the substantive domain of the sociology of health and health care was initially and has remained philosophical and theoretical. The present volume has provided an opportunity to pull together strands in my thinking that straddle what are often even now seen and treated as discrete discourses: philosophically grounded theory on the one hand, and substantive research on the other. Doubtless I have fallen short of my aspirations, but my overriding aim has been to put together a critical account of sociology's contribution to our understanding of health and health care in modern societies like Britain. Why 'critical'? It is an adjective that I deploy quite readily having learned much from Jurgen Habermas's late-Frankfurt School *critical* theory and Roy Bhaskar's *critical* realism. What my and their usages have in common is a commitment not only to achieving understanding, or even explaining, but to an 'active' publicly oriented sociology beyond the artificial constraints of Hume's 'is-ought' dichotomy.

Several of the chapters are given over to or incorporate explications of dense philosophical and theoretical arguments developed by Habermas, Bhaskar and others. I have considered myself bound, however, by a stricture or two. The first and most important one for me is that my sociology is geared to throwing such light on the interrelations between society and health as allows people to see a short way ahead. To this end, my more abstruse digressions are subordinated to the sociological project as I see it. While I consider it important to represent others' arguments faithfully, my paramount concern is with *sociology, health and health care. Getting a credible grasp of how things are, why they are as they are and what might be done to change them for the better trumps all else*. This is most salient in relation to Bhaskar's dialectical critical realism (or DCR). A development well beyond his basic critical realism (BCR), DCR is notoriously resistant to exegesis. But this matters less to me here than DCR's potential to deepen, underpin and reinvigorate the sociological project. I do not hesitate to learn lessons from Bhaskar's BCR and DCR that might not have been intended; that is, I am faithful to a point, but not above all else.

My second stricture is that I regard sociology both as irreducible 'downwards' towards psychology, biology and beyond, or 'upwards' towards anthropology and beyond. And yet, sociology can only ever contribute partially to our understanding, explanations of and interventions in the field of health and health care. Sociologists can never wrap things up. Acknowledging my own limitations, I nevertheless attempt in this book to address the concept of *interdisciplinarity* in ways that help contextualize the sociological project.

Third, this book comes under the rubric of what I call *meta-reflection*. By this I mean that it is a contribution that draws on a now vast body of empirical research and offers a theoretical synthesis. One largely unintended consequence of the neo-liberalization of British and other universities is a rapid turnaround of research outputs, be they empirical studies or theoretical or conceptual explorations. Meta-reflection has become in my view an increasingly valuable but neglected enterprise. To take a single example, and one that will be revisited in detail in later chapters, there is almost a superfluity of research documenting health inequalities in and between nation states. But much of it is embedded in a socio-epidemiological (*not* a quantitative sociological) paradigm. It follows that it bears the stamp of the kind of positivism represented in J.S. Mills's nineteenth-century canons of scientific enquiry and long since exposed for the pseudo-science it is. It is no longer credible to rely on statistical associations thrown up by 'variable analysis'. Nor is it just the positivistic *analysis* that it at fault. As symbolic interactionist Blumer noted long ago, social phenomena do not readily admit to division into chunks or *variables*. If this seems too dismissive of extant socio-epidemiological data, then I should add that they remain 'grist to the mill' for sociologists. Enter critical realism.

In the first chapter, I trace changing historical patterns of disease and mortality over time and raise the ever-present issue of social and health inequalities. The agenda-shifting Black Report of 1980 is discussed in his connection, as are research findings from socio-epidemiological studies deploying socioeconomic proxies for social class. While acknowledging that such studies supply clues for a sociology oriented – as I maintain it should be – to explanation, I offer a critique of the positivist methods owing much to Hume and J.S. Mill and still put to use by sociologists interested in examining health inequalities. The message here is that we should expect, and can deliver, more from a sociological engagement with health inequalities.

Chapter 2 is given over to critical expositions, and brief assessments, of sociology's main schools of thought and their relevance to the sociology of health generally and to the sociology of health inequalities in particular. The perspectives considered are structural-functionalism; interactionism; phenomenology and ethnomethodology; social constructionism; post-structuralism and postmodernism; conflict and critical theory; and feminist, post-colonial and disability theory. The lessons learned from these discussions is that each of these non- or post-positivist perspectives has much to teach; that their questions and answers often overlap; and that no perspective, nor indeed sociology in its entirety, should aspire to wraps things up.

In Chapter 3, Bhaskar's philosophy of critical realism is introduced. The focus in the first part is on his *basic* critical realism. It is argued that this approach has a threefold return: it overcomes what he calls the 'epistemic fallacy' – that is, reducing what exists to what we can know of what exists – and provides an ontology of objects, powers/mechanisms and tendencies without falling into the trap of reductionism; it offers a viable alternative to positivism in its multiple guises; and it announces and commits to methodological rigour in a (dynamic and 'messy') open society. In the second part, I outline what I contend are the main and compelling features of post-1970s financial capitalism. In the final part, I spell out the relevance of this macro-sociological analysis for understanding and explaining health inequalities and the present 'selling off' of the English National Health Service (NHS) to for-profit providers. The core concepts and roles of the novel class/command dynamic of financial capitalism and of asset flows pertinent for health and longevity are defined.

Chapter 4 introduces another critical realist, Margaret Archer. Her approach to the structure/agency issue and her theories of morphogenesis, morphogentic cycles and reflexivity are drawn upon to throw further light on financial capitalism and to show how agency is socially structured, if never socially determined. Developing her idea of reflexive 'internal conversations', I introduce two ideal types of special salience for health inequalities: the *focused autonomous reflexive* and the *vulnerable fractured reflexive*. The former are instrumental in the production and reproduction of health inequalities, the latter most at risk of sickness and premature mortality. Four middle-range theories that help explain the social structuring of agency that impacts on health are outlined: *effort/reward imbalance, relative risk aversion, ego adjustment* and *activity reinforcement.*

In the fifth chapter, I offer an abbreviated exposition of Bhaskar's *dialectical* critical realism. Recognising that the challenge here is to show just *how* his esoteric and dense philosophical treatise has something to offer the sociological project, I concentrate on the ideas of *absence* and *negating negation*. Absence is a ripple on the ocean of being. The query 'what is absent from the extant sociology of health inequalities?' admits, I suggest, of a number of significant answers. One answer is pursued in some detail: a theory of what Bhaskar calls 'power 2 relations'. In other words, our sociology of health inequalities is a sociology reconciled to avoiding the causal force of social structures in general and class (and class struggle) in particular. A renewal via the absenting of absence and of 'constraining ills' is commended.

Chapter 6 draws on some of the perspectives from chapter two, plus others (notably Zizek, Ritzer, Bauman, Castells and Tyler), to offer a characterisation of the *fractured society* that financial capitalism has spawned. The analysis that follows is framed by social disintegration, class as an absent presence, McDonaldisation as end-stage control, surplus cultural liquidity, flows and superhubs and the weaponising of stigma. The conclusion to this chapter pulls together multiple and diverse threads to articulate what I take to be a genuinely sociological theory of health inequalities.

In Chapter 7, consideration is given to the key questions: 'what to do?'/'how best to tackle health inequalities?' How might a transformative politics promote the kind of changes that might prove effective? If Streeck is right, capitalism might be on its last legs, although any post-capitalist future remains a matter of speculation; nor indeed should its powers of self-preservation be under-estimated. Forces conducive to social transformation/emancipation are perused, and a new and pro-change ideal type – that of the *dedicated meta-reflexive* – introduced. Factors lending themselves to: (a) the status quo and (b) change are reviewed. Reference is then made to 'future studies' and an argument made, drawing on Urry's pioneering work, that sociology's reach should extend to absenting both absence and constraining ills. I argue that promulgating 'concrete utopias', via a programme of *permanent reform*, might ease in change conducive to reducing health inequalities. I cite the contribution of the journalist Paul Mason here.

In the final chapter, the sociological project I advocate is summarised. This is rooted in what Habermas called *lifeworld rationalisation*. Why else, I ask rhetorically but pointedly, do we do sociology? What follows amounts to a sociological manifesto for a twenty-first century sociology in general, and for a sociology of health inequalities in particular. The role of each of *six sociologies* (professional, policy, critical, public, foresight and action) is appraised, and the salience of foresight and action sociology is highlighted. The volume concludes with items that might comprise a provisional agenda for a credible, effective and future-oriented *sociology* of health inequalities, plus a comment or two on the book's limitations.

Part I

1 Health as a social lens

It will be obvious to anyone who as much as sneaks a look at this book's title that it is premised on the notion that an understanding of a society is crucial if we are to grasp the health of its population. It is a notion that has left sociology and entered that precarious world of common sense. The health and life expectancy of populations, groups and individuals, contemporary wisdom acknowledges, are at least in part a function of social location, circumstances and learned or imitated behaviours. Healers and the institutions through which they ply their wares are no less socially anchored. A little more reflection may be required, however, to appreciate that the health of a people and the mode of delivery of any system of treatment and care also offers insight into a society. In this opening chapter, I try to show why health is a *social lens* as well as a social product. It is a chapter of two parts, the first outlining a standard account of changes in health and, in particular, longevity over time, the second interrogating this account.

Health, death and some parameters

No single definition of 'being healthy' spans the vagaries of time and space. Indeed, the concept has a peculiarly modern ring to it. Even what we would understand as 'threats to health' do not travel well. It is a modern conceit, in other words, to presume that 'our' modern – and occidental – concepts and discourses reach back beyond late-eighteenth century Europe or extend to developing societies, let alone deep to the origins of human sociability amongst nomadic hunter-gathering clusters prior to the Neolithic revolution from around 8,000 to 3,000 BC.

Unsurprisingly, death travels better: it is one thing to debate health status, wellbeing and quality of life, quite another to reflect on the finitude of the human lifespan on Earth. On the basis of analyses of surviving artefacts, it has been suggested that the expectation of life at birth for hunter-gatherers eking out a life-course of hardship, unpredictability and subsistence probably did not much exceed 20 years or so. This is naturally a 'guesstimate'. And those who made it through the perilous initial weeks, months and years of infancy and childhood doubtless added on a good few more years. How does this compare with the more accurate data available in subsequent social formations?

There is a view that life expectancy at birth actually decreased prior to the Neolithic revolution as climate change affected diet (Roberts & Cox, 2003). What is certainly striking is that it increased so slowly over such a long period after the Neolithic revolution. As humans settled and tamed the land, turned to agriculture, established and patrolled their boundaries as newborn nation states and pioneered industrial production, the number of years the newborn could expect to live crept up at a snail's pace. But it bears repetition that surviving childbirth and infancy has *always* been critical. Historian Ian Mortimer (2014: 3) puts it well in his study of change from 1000 to 2000:

> even in the Middle Ages, some men and women lived to 90 years of age or more. St Gilbert of Sempringham died in 1189 at the age of 106; Sir John de Sully died in 1387 at 105. Very few people today live any longer than that. True, there were comparatively few octogenerians in the Middle Ages – 50 per cent of babies did not even reach adulthood – but in terms of the maximum lifespan possible, there was little change across the whole millennium.

When Victoria ascended the throne in the first country to industrialise, imperial and liberal capitalist *Great* Britain, life expectancy at birth was only around 40 years (a year or two more for women than men). Given that in this same country we now anticipate living approximately 80 years (77 for men, 81 for women), it follows that there has been an extraordinary increase in life expectancy at birth in less than two centuries. But Britain here represents the developed, prosperous, imperialist West. Elsewhere across the twenty-first century globe, life expectancy at birth still languishes: in 'developing' Ethiopia it is 41 for men and 43 for women, and in Sierra Leone 33 for men and 35 for women.

So, if the years one might reasonably expect to live have taken off in nation states like Britain, this is certainly far from the case in most developing countries. Three questions might be posed here. The first and obvious one is: 'why this dramatic change in many developed nations?'; the second is: 'why has this change not been echoed in developing nations?'; and the third is: 'what is it that comparative national statistics on life expectancy at birth *are not telling us*?'. No answer to any of these questions is beyond dispute. Nor is this simply a function of the prudent scientific admission of 'fallibilism', namely, the recognition that one might at some future point be proven mistaken about *anything or everything*.

The first query has been comprehensively addressed and argued over. In the pre-agricultural era of the hunter-gathers, it is probable that many deaths resulted from malnutrition, a plethora of environmental hazards and violent conflict. Between 8,000 and 3,000 BC, however, new patterns of sociality emerged. Table One maps these modes of sociality from the time of the Neolithic revolution to the present (Table 1.1).

Table 1.1 A Chronology of Human Social Formations

From the beginning of the Neolithic revolution, occurring from 8,000 to 3,000 BC, sociopolitical evolution encompassed four principal stages:

1 *Bands* – small nomadic groups of up to a dozen hunter-gatherers; democratic and egalitarian (close to Marx's 'primitive communism').
2 *Tribes* – similar to bands except more committed to horticulture and pastoralism; 'segmentary societies' comprising autonomous villages.
3 *Chiefdoms* – autonomous political units under permanent control of paramount chief, central government with hereditary, hierarchical status arrangements; 'rank societies'.
4 *States* – autonomous political units; centralised government supported by monopoly of violence; large dense populations characterised by stratification and inequality.

3,000 BC witnessed the birth of fully fledged agrarian states, displaying a number of core characteristics and remaining the predominant form of social organization until around 1450 AD. These core characteristics can be summarised as follows:

• a division of labour between a small landowning (or controlling) nobility and a large peasantry; this was an exploitative division backed by military force.
• the noble-peasant relationship provided the principal axis in agrarian societies: it was a relationship based on production-for-use rather than production-for-exchange.
• differences of interest between nobles and peasants, but not overt 'class struggle'.
• societies held together not by consensus but by military force.
• societies relatively static and unchanging: there was a 4,500-year incubation period prior to the advent of capitalist states.

The transition to capitalism took place in the 'long sixteenth century', that is, between 1450 and 1640. Marx saw this transition as of major significance, noting three vital characteristics of the new capitalist system:

• private ownership of the means of production by the bourgeoisie.
• the existence of wage-labour as the basis of production.
• the profit motive and long-term accumulation of capital as the driving aim of production.

It is customary to discern reasonably distinct stages of capitalism. Thus a transition to 'merchant capitalism' is typically dates from 1450 to 1640, followed by a period of consolidation and solidification, characterised by slow, steady growth between 1640 and 1760. 1760 is often cited as a marker for a switch to 'industrial capitalism', which is itself often divided into stages:

1 *Early industrial*, 1760–1830: textile manufacturing dominated by Britain.
2 *Liberal*, 1830–1870: railroads and iron dominated by Britain and later the USA.
3 *Liberal/Early Fordist*, 1870-WW1: steel and organic chemistry, with the emergence of new industries based on producing and using electrical machinery, dominated by the USA and Germany.
4 *Late Fordist/Welfare*, WW1–1970: automobiles and petrochemicals, dominated by the USA.
5 *Financial*, 1970 onwards: electronics, information and biotechnology, plus global finance, dominated by the USA, also Japan and Western Europe.

Sociologists tend to be more open to *periodization* than are the more Whiggish of historians, but, setting finer or philosophical controversies aside for the moment, the periodization outlined in the table allows for a framing, mapping and contextualizing of sociopolitical change over time. It offers a useful broad-brush scoping of our past useful for present purposes.

The switch to full-blown agricultural states as bands, tribes and chiefdoms became more peripheral after 3,000 BC impacted heavily on the major causes of death. Agriculture required permanent settlement. The development of cereals permitted more mouths to be fed, in the process supporting higher population densities, but also, paradoxically, narrowed and diminished people's diet and immunity to infection. So, unbeknown to inhabitants of all strata, agricultural states delivered novel threats to people's health in the guise of several potent infectious diseases. Nor were there any sanitary arrangements, the significance of which was also unknown. This led to the contamination of water supplies.

With the advantage of hindsight, the major infectious diseases showed four modes of transmission: (a) *airborne* (like tuberculosis); (b) *waterborne* (like cholera); (c) *food-borne* (like dysentery); and (d) *vector-borne* (like plague and malaria). The infamous plague, the Black Death of 1348, decimated the population of England and of Europe as a whole, accounting for one-quarter of its population. It made its last appearance in Britain in 1665 but died out thereafter; it was spread by fleas carried by black rats and lost its potency as black rats were displaced by their brown brethren, the latter being less prone to infest human settlements (Fitzpatrick & Speed, 2018).

The thesis that the rapid acceleration of longevity after the mid-nineteenth century in Britain was down to the diminishing impact of the infectious diseases has a solid epidemiological pedigree (although it should be noted that these diseases did not all decline simultaneously). Fitzpatrick and Chandola (2000: 102) summarise:

> the declining significance of infectious diseases was the single main reason for the dramatic increase in life expectancy ... Conversely, the main reason for the increase in heart disease, strokes and cancer has been that individuals were increasingly likely to reach the older ages at which these diseases typically, although not exclusively, occur.

It should be noted that improvements in mortality occurred *at different times for different age groups*. In Britain, the first marked improvement occurred in the 5–24 age group around 1860. Infant mortality fell steadily from 1900 with conspicuous accelerations during the early and late years of postwar welfare capitalism: *in 1900, one-quarter of all deaths in the population occurred in the first year of life, but by the end of the century this had declined to 1%*. Mortality rates for the 15–44 age group improved in the course of the twentieth century, although with interruptions from the influenza epidemic of 1918 and for the two world wars. Improvements for those aged 45–54 also started at the beginning of the century; for those aged 55–74, mortality declined from the 1920s; for those aged over 74, the decline began in the years after the second world war. For older age groups, the most marked improvements in mortality have taken place since the 1970s (Fitzpatrick & Chandola, 2000; Scambler, 2002).

By the mid-twentieth century, the so-called degenerative diseases like cancer and cardiovascular disease had taken over as the major causes of death. Moreover, Britain was unexceptional: mercantilist-to-capitalist industrialization, whenever and wherever found, seemed somehow to precipitate this shift. McKeown (1979) was the research pioneer. He challenged the obvious inference that scientific advance had allowed medicine to deliver on its more extravagant and newly 'professionised' promises.

A number of possible causes for the general displacement of the infectious diseases as the major causes of death have been mooted, apart that is from scientific and medical advancement and intervention. These fall into three categories: (a) a decline in the virulence of the organisms responsible for the diseases; (b) a reduction in human exposure to the infectious organisms (e.g. through reduced contamination of supplies of water and food); (c) an enhanced genetic human resistance to infection due to Darwinian selection processes; and (d) an increased human resistance to infection via improved nutrition and general fitness that (i) reduced the probability of being infected and/or (ii) increased the chances of recovery from infection. It is not of course simply a matter of picking out one from (a) to (d). No more can it be assumed that (a) to (d) can be prioritised across all the major infectious diseases or all societies. In fact, most commentators discount the salience of (a) and (c) in Britain on the dual grounds that the decline across the infectious diseases occurred *over too short a period of time* and *across all the major diseases*. This leaves (b) and (d).

The evidence in favour of (d), in particular the improved nutritional intake resulting from innovative agricultural techniques and the speedier and more efficient transportation of produce under liberal capitalism, seems indubitable. No less important, the nineteenth century as a whole witnessed an unprecedented increase in real wages and the standard of living in Britain. As Fitzpatrick & Speed (2018) remark, (d) was for McKeown (1979) underpinned by evidence from the developing world: he cited a World Health Organization (WHO) report that one-half to three-quarters of all recorded deaths of infants and young children could be attributed to a combination of malnutrition and infection. This does not mean, however, that (b) is insignificant.

(b), or reduced exposure to infection, played its role too. The iconic case is John Snow's experimental or proto-epidemiological removal of a pump handle in London's Soho, affirming cholera's status as a waterborne disease. This initiative epitomises the emergence in the nineteenth century of a novel and powerful public health movement. Moves were made to prevent the contamination of supplies of drinking water by sewage (gastroenteric diseases were under control by the beginning of the twentieth century, dramatically impacting on infant mortality); and the sterilization of milk and its more hygienic transportation in particular, and improved food hygiene in general, comprised another environmental shift that lent itself to the decline in infectious disease mortality (Fitzpatrick & Speed, 2018).

McKeown and his public health disciples have not had it all their own way however. While it must be accepted that environmental factors were critical for the historically 'recent' extension in longevity, at least in developed nations, there are those who trace this back and attribute causal priority to Adam Smith's 'invisible hand' of capitalism. They are right to look for signs rather than symptoms, I shall argue later, but the appropriate diagnosis alludes them.

The ugly intrusion of inequality

Thus far, it has been noted that the human lifespan has increased in conjunction with inevitably complex and dynamic processes of social change, leading from nomadic hunter-gatherer groups via agricultural settlements and states to more highly differentiated industrial, even post-industrial, social formations. Changed environmental, social and individual circumstances impacted not only on how long people lived but on which diseases most threatened their survival. But apart from briefly recording a stark gap between the rates of morality of developed and developing societies, no mention has been made of the salience of inequality.

As Therborn (2014) has insisted, the equality/inequality dichotomy carries a normative element: equality is positive, inequality negative. In sociological terms, negative states of inequality have conventionally been linked to social stratification, or the hierarchical ranking found in one guise or another in virtually all societies since 'primitive' hunter-gatherer communities and their immediate progeny. For Marx, unifying themes link historical systems of stratification; for others, like Weber, such systems are multi-dimensional and variable. For now, it is enough to explore in preliminary fashion the extent to which in stratified social formations those occupying the higher strata tend to live longer than those languishing in the lower strata.

It is one thing to claim that historically the rich and powerful in the uppermost stratum have tended to live longer than the poor and powerless in the lowest stratum, and quite another to assert that longevity has increased *stratum-by-stratum* across hierarchic social formations. Contingency often intervenes. For example, the Black Death killed the monks and clergy who administered to the sick before decimating the poorer labouring classes. Moreover, reliable evidence is hard to come by, at least until the Victorian era in Britain.

Coinciding with the heyday of the infectious diseases around the middle of the nineteenth century there emerged – crossing the channel from France – statistical initiatives to document changing social conditions. The collation of statistics was boosted with the passage of the Registration Act in 1836, which for the first time required the registration of births, marriages and deaths (plus cause of death). Statistician William Farr, who spent 40 years working for the Registrar General, the bureaucratic apparatus established to implement the Registration Act, pioneered the tabulation of mortality rates and life tables disaggregated by occupational status and place of residence (Eyler, 1979). Farr's work made it possible to show more clearly and precisely how the greatest burden of disease fell on the poor and labouring or working class.

Chadwick's *Report on the Sanitary Condition of the Labouring Population of Great Britain* in 1842 drew on Farr's painstaking innovations to document the level of health inequality. In Manchester, the average age of death for 'professional persons and gentry and their families' was 38, for 'tradesmen and their families' 20 and for 'mechanics, labourers and their families' 17 (1842: 223). These dramatic figures reflect a very high rate of infant mortality: amongst Manchester's working class, over half (57%) of deaths occurred under the age of five (1842: 224). Not that Chadwick had anything much to say about poverty as a cause of premature deaths. In fact, his understandable but limiting fixation on sanitation and general prejudice in favour of the Poor Law effectively precluded him from taking poverty seriously (as his vigorous exchange of letters with Farr at the time testifies). As we shall see later, it was left to the likes of Virchow (Taylor & Rieger, 1985) and Engels (1999) to correct this myopia (Scambler, 2012a).

Health inequalities in contemporary capitalism

What are we to make of health inequalities in Britain more than a century and half after the early interventions of Chadwick, Farr and Engels? To what extent does poverty: (a) persist and (b) impact on health? The methodological obstacles to tracking changes should not be underestimated: populations sampled and measures of position and circumstance deployed have often been revised since the mid-nineteenth century (Bartley, 2016). But certainly, health inequalities have not gone away. It was the 'Black Report' that crystallised attention by offering a state-of-the-art synopsis and set of recommendations for policy change pertinent for the era of what I shall hereafter call 'financial capitalism' (Black, 1982). This Report drew on health data from the Registrar General dating back to the second quarter of the nineteenth century. What these data suggested was that health and longevity declined with what might best be called occupational prestige or status. There was an early hint too of a general stratum-by-stratum decline of the kind mooted above and which has since become known as the 'social gradient'.

In their summation of the evidence, Black and his colleagues emphasised the causal significance of 'materialist' or social structural factors for health and life expectancy. These were indicative of people's generalised standard of living and included 'relative poverty' (which had by then largely displaced 'absolute poverty'). Black and associates accorded them top priority in a ranking of four contributors. Second came 'cultural' or 'behavioural' factors like smoking, excessive drinking, poor diet and overly sedentary lifestyles. There was mention, third, of 'social selection', in recognition that poor health can itself result in declining occupational status, as is commonly found in transnational studies of schizophrenia for example. Lastly, the importance of precise measurement was noted, although the hypothesis that the statistical association between occupational status and health was 'artefactual' was rejected.

The Black Report proved politically contentious. Commissioned by Callaghan's Labour government in the mid-1970s it saw the light of day during Thatcher's post-1979 Conservative regime. Its emphasis on materialist or social structural factors sat uncomfortably with the neophyte Health Minister Patrick Jenkin, who said as much in a grudging foreword. Through the 1980s and beyond, right-of-centre governments made an ideological decision to accent cultural or behavioural over materialist or social structural factors, which allowed them to transfer responsibility for health and longevity from government to the individual.

The Black Report proved a catalyst for researchers. It was to have progeny in the form of the Acheson Report (1998) and the Marmot Review (2010). Each of these reaffirmed the continuing existence of (a) health inequalities, and (b) a social gradient. What each also bore testimony to was a deepening of health inequalities through the era of financial capitalism. So what is the present state of play? In 2001 the Registrar General's schema, once aptly characterised as more blunderbuss than carefully calibrated instrument, was displaced by the National Statistics Socio-Economic Classification (NS-SEC). While the Registrar General's schema was based on an under-researched and changeable sense of occupational prestige, NS-SEC factored in not only occupational status but other dimensions of employment like job security, autonomy, opportunity and so on. Table 1.2 gives an outline of each of these classifications. Each has been imprudently considered a proxy for social class, a contentious issue we return to in detail later in this volume.

Table 1.3 records life expectancy at birth by gender and the Registrar General's classification of occupational status during financial capitalism. Table 1.4 gives age-standardised mortality rates by gender and NS-SEC for adults aged between 25 and 64 for the years 2001, 2005 and 2010.

What do these data tell us? Table 1.3 suggests that while life expectancy at birth improved across all occupational statuses during financial capitalism, it did so more for those in higher than in lower strata. In other words, the already advantaged have built on their advantage. Table 1.3, focusing on differential death rates rather than life expectancy, affirms via the more refined

Table 1.2 Registrar General's Classification and NS-SEC

Registrar general		NS-SEC	
I	Professional	1	Higher managerial/professional
II	Intermediate	2	Lower managerial/professional
IIIa	Skilled non-manual	3	Intermediate
IIIb	Skilled manual	4	Small employers/self-employed
IV	Semi-skilled manual	5	Lower supervisory
V	Unskilled manual	6	Semi-routine
		7	Routine

Sources: I-IIIa Non-manual or 'middle class'; IIIb-V Manual or 'working class'

Table 1.3 Life Expectancy at Birth by Gender and RG Occupational Status

Occupational status	1972–1976		1987–1991		2002–2005	
	Males	Females	Males	Females	Males	Females
I	71.9	79.0	76.2	81.1	80.0	85.1
II	71.9	77.1	75.0	80.7	79.4	83.2
IIIN	69.5	78.3	74.4	80.0	78.4	82.4
IIIM	70.0	75.2	72.7	77.9	76.5	80.5
IV	68.3	75.3	70.8	77.4	75.7	79.9
V	66.5	74.2	68.7	76.6	72.7	78.1
Non-manual (I-IIIN)	71.2	77.7	75.0	80.4	79.2	82.9
Manual (IIIM-V)	69.1	75.2	71.7	77.5	75.9	80.0
All	69.3	75.3	72.6	78.3	77.0	81.1

Source: ONS (2007)

device of NS-SEC that although death rates have declined for all strata, the rate of decline has been significantly more rapid amongst the highest than amongst the lowest through the 'noughties'. Moreover, these trends and this pattern hold for morbidity as well as for mortality. Health inequalities, it seems, are increasing in financial capitalism (see Nettleton, 2013).

Since the Black Report, there has been some movement in explanatory models for health inequalities. If material or social structural factors have held their ground, ideological reinterpretations aside, there is a growing reluctance to 'separate them off' from cultural or behavioural factors. There is increasing evidence, the argument runs, that our cultural scripts and behaviours are shaped by – even a function of – the material resources available to us. Is it any wonder that hard-up single mums buy cheaper food and smoke? This elides into another newer model that emphasises 'psychosocial pathways' from resources to behaviours (via culture). Material inequality leads to social fragmentation and a loss of reciprocity and trust in others that issues in enhanced stress levels and vulnerability to disease. Social selection has become more peripheral; and better measurement has led to a sharper, not a blunter, calculation of the extent and growth of health inequalities.

Table 1.4 Age-Standardised Mortality Rates by Gender and NS-SEC for Adults
         Aged 25–64 in 2001, 2005 and 2010

	Rate per 100,000 people		
	2001	*2005*	*2010*
Males			
Higher managerial/professional	178	147	128
Lower managerial/professional	280	249	210
Intermediate	296	287	253
Self-employed	339	307	278
Lower supervisory	373	339	317
Semi-routine	465	420	399
Routine	564	514	458
Females			
Higher managerial/professional	105	94	80
Lower managerial/professional	145	131	122
Intermediate	155	157	156
Self-employed	180	167	153
Lower supervisory	205	184	186
Semi-routine	225	244	230
Routine	318	285	287

Source: See ONS (2012)

   In an influential and public intervention, epidemiologists Wilkinson and
Pickett (2009) have contended that it is the psychosocial pathways from differential material resources (in their contribution, incomes) to behaviours
that offer the optimal focus for a theory of health inequalities. In a contro-
versial and contested summation of inter- and intra-national statistics, they
purport to show that although the affluence of modern capitalism has been
accompanied by increases in life expectancy, there is a point beyond which
a nation's or area's growing affluence ceases to show a generalised return
in terms of longevity. At this point, it is no longer growing affluence per se
that is key but the *distribution of material resources.* In a nutshell, rich *equal*
nations or areas have superior life expectancies to rich *unequal* nations or
areas. Among developed societies, this thesis suggests, the extent of material
equality is a critical component of any credible social theory of health inequalities (see Dorling, 2013).
   These are the conclusions of social epidemiology not of sociology (Scambler,
2012a). For now, what they do is buttress the historical contention that a
person's social position partly determines his or her life-chances, health and
longevity. Relative poverty, the modern substitute for the absolute poverty
rampant into Victorian times, 'somehow or other' occasions poor health
and kills prematurely. It is certainly unfortunate to be born – and remain –
of low social standing.
   So what do the sections comprising this opening chapter so far add up to?
There seems little doubt about the following:

- how long people live and the predominant threats to their health and longevity have varied historically (and are likely to continue to do so);
- there occurred a quite dramatic increase in life expectancy in mid- to late-nineteenth century Britain;
- this increase in life expectancy was facilitated initially by public health and later by medical interventions that witnessed a displacement of infectious by chronic or long-term diseases as the major life-takers;
- there is a strong case for regarding (absolute and subsequently relative) poverty as an enduring contributor to poor health and premature death;
- material deprivation is not the only factor predisposing to poor health/ longevity;
- while there is no longer a consensus that women experience higher rates of morbidity than men, in most societies they tend to outlive men.

There are two significant riders to append to these bullet points. The first is that occupational class and gender both come simultaneously into play when we assess the social determinants of health and longevity. To these we might add a range of other factors, ethnicity being an obvious one. And second, there is a difference between seeing factors like occupational class and gender as *variables* and envisioning them as *social structures* or *relations*. And this remark in particular should and will lead to a critical revisiting of our narrative.

From on-the-surface to beneath-the-surface: a critique

Problems with positivism

Social epidemiology represents a pure, and too much quantitative sociology an impure, form of *positivism*, and this is the key that unlocks my critique of the argument to this point. Positivism has its roots in a philosophy of empiricism hinted at long ago in the pioneering writings of the pre-Socratics and consolidated in the later epistemologies of Locke, Berkeley and Hume. Of these 'British empiricists', Hume is the pivotal figure for present purposes. It is sufficient to focus here on his account of causality and constant conjunctions found in his *Treatise of Hunan Nature*, published in 1739/1740. It seemed for Hume that if we are asked for our evidence that A is the cause of B, the only possible answer is that A and B have been constantly conjoined in the past. This does not prove that they are invariably associated. The only recourse then left to us is to admit the 'psychological' origins of our inferences: 'all our reasonings concerning causes and effects', Hume asserts, 'are derived from nothing but custom'. So the connection between A and B consists in the fact that we cannot help – psychologically, not logically – under certain circumstances having certain expectations. If we are asked to justify causal inferences, all we can do is describe how we think.

Hume's thesis haunts as well as informs positivist approaches, past and present. Comte's promotion of a positivist science of society in his *Cours de Philosophe Positive*, issued in six volumes between 1830 and 1842, proved a catalyst. J.S. Mill, less interested in Comte's sociology than in nailing a credible methodology for social science, added a refinement that is also a comment on Hume. For him the cause of any event is a set of conditions or factors that, taken together, constitute a sufficient condition for it; his 'sets of conditions' replace Hume's single events. Mill developed an inductive model of social science from a perspective of an uncompromising methodological individualism inimical to Comte. He spelled out a series of canons or procedures of 'agreement', 'difference', 'residues' and 'concomitant variation' for testing hypotheses or causal relations. 'Mill's' canons will strike an immediate chord with authors and disciples of the bread-and-butter analyses of social epidemiology and epidemiologically oriented sociology whose findings and conclusions were summarised earlier.

Two principles underpin 'Mill's' 'eliminative induction': (a) that nothing which was absent when an event occurred could be its cause; and (b) that nothing which was present when an event failed to occur could be its cause. Mill did not distinguish between necessary and sufficient conditions – in fact, by 'cause' he understood sufficient condition not necessary condition – but his canons are perhaps most effectively explicated using this terminology.

His method of agreement states that if two or more instances of the phenomenon under investigation have only one circumstance in common, the circumstance in which alone all the instances agree is the cause (or effect) of the given phenomenon. In brief, this is a method designed to determine possible necessary conditions by elimination. The method of difference states that if an instance in which the phenomenon under investigation occurs and an instance in which it does not occur have every circumstance in common save one, that one occurring only in the former, the circumstance in which alone the two instances differ is the effect or the cause of the phenomenon. This is a method for determining possible sufficient conditions by elimination. Mill allows too for a joint method of agreement and difference.

The method of residues asserts that if known causes cannot account for a phenomenon, it is necessary to seek a cause elsewhere: there must be some residual factor that is not known and/or has not been taken into account. It is a method that hinges on deduction rather than induction. The method of concomitant variation states that whatever phenomenon varies in any manner whenever another phenomenon varies in some particular manner is either a cause or an effect of that phenomenon or is connected with it through some fact of causation. It is a method to be deployed, in other words, when a given factor cannot be removed, rendering the method of difference redundant.

Mill's argument has been refined many times over by social statisticians, but his canons are more illuminative of current positivistic sociological practice than many of their more 'sophisticated' successors. Consider the following triad, each of which trades on Hume's regularity theory of causation:

1   the *deductive nomological* model associated with Hempel, in which premises, statements of general laws and statements of antecedent conditions (the *explanans*) permit the deduction of a conclusion, a statement describing the event to be explained (the *explanandum*).
2   the *inductive-statistical* model, in which the statements of general laws in the deductive-nomological model give way to probabilistic or statistical generalizations, and the relationship between premises and conclusion is one of inductive probability not deductive necessity.
3   the *hypothetico-deductive* model devised by Popper (and interpreted here as a variant of positivism), in which the emphasis is placed not on (indecisively) confirming a conjecture or theory but on (decisively) falsifying it by a counter-observation.

What is wrong with the positivism of Mill and his progeny? I have previously differentiated between three types of positivistic investigation in the sociology of health and health care (Scambler, 2002). Two of these can be defended. The first I called *accounting*, which refers to the collection and/or collation of data to discern social patterns of behaviour and circumstance, often via the deployment of cross-sectional surveys of large populations. Accounting describes. The second I called *advising*, which refers to a subset of investigations of social patterns of behaviour and circumstance *designed to steer policy and its implementation*. For advising, *prediction can be key*, especially in the event of a rapidly spreading epidemic, for example. In much clinical and public health research, it is prediction that has to be prioritised when urgent intervention is required; explanation must needs wait, though when it arrives its input is likely to be corrective and inestimable.

It is the third type of positivism – *predicting/explaining* – that is more problematic. Studies oriented to predicting/explaining aim not merely to identify social patterns of behaviour and circumstance but to explain them; and for the positivist, *explaining and predicting are two sides of the same coin*. The spirit of Mill lives on in such investigations, which, nowadays, tend to follow the inductive-statistical model (Hempel's model having been largely rejected, and Popper's largely untried). In his *Economics and Reality*, Lawson (1997: 19) writes:

if particular knowledge is restricted to atomistic events given in experience, the only possibility for general, including scientific, knowledge is the elaboration of patterns of association of these events. It is thus such constant event patterns, or regularities of the form 'whenever event X then event Y', that constitute the Humean or positivist account of causal laws.

Lawson goes on to argue that the world is not composed merely of experience and events, but also of underlying 'mechanisms' that exist whether or not detected and that shape or facilitate events. This is so, he maintains, for social as well as natural science. Moreover – a crucial point – events are typically (a) 'unsynchronised' with the mechanisms that shape them; and (b) 'conjointly determined by various, perhaps countervailing influences so that the governing causes, though necessarily "appearing" through, or in, events can rarely be read straight off'. In other words, the 'true' objects of sociological enquiry – that is, mechanisms like class, gender, ethnicity and so on – only manifest themselves in 'open systems' where 'constant event patterns' or 'regularities' of the kind pursued by positivists rarely, if ever, obtain. We have seen that much of the research reported thus far is of this type.

Two remarks are in order at this juncture. First, this compelling but attenuated critique of positivism, courtesy of Lawson, will be the subject of progressive elaboration in subsequent chapters: it offers a tantalizing glimpse of what (basic) critical realism promises. And second, it needs to be stressed that historical and current positivistic research alike deliver what Lawson terms 'demi-regularities' (or 'demi-regs'), which fuel genuine sociological enquiry. Epidemiologists and quantitative sociologists accepting of Mill's canons *nevertheless* provide us with useful data. It is just that these data are more suggestive and less decisive than they would have us believe.

Beyond Hume's 'is/ought' dichotomy

These paragraphs pick up on a point by Therborn cited earlier: equality is commended, inequality condemned. But we should first return to Hume. Hume's argument is seductive. You simply cannot, he asserted, infer an 'ought' from an 'is'. No matter how much data exist on what 'is' the case, no translation into what 'ought' to be the case is permitted. But matters are surely more complex. Sociology necessarily reaches out to the historical constructions of generations of people whose actions were motivated by ideas that might or might not have been in their interests. To draw on a notion of Archer's (1995), people's natal, 'involuntary' placement in an established hierarchical order can lead them to act against their interests, mistakenly or unawares. Creaven (2007: 16) clarifies:

> powerholders and superordinate groups have both vested interests and the institutional and cultural capacities to disseminate their own self-justificatory beliefs across the rest of society, to misinterpret unegalitarian social relations as in the interests of everyone, or to justify publicly their own oppressive or exploitative institutions in the eyes of the downtrodden or subordinate.

If it is accepted (a) that people's interpretations of the world are part and parcel of 'social reality', and (b) that these interpretations can be partial, imprecise or simply wrong, then it is surely a task of the sociologist to reveal the ways in which such interpretations are problematic and why this is the case. Occasionally these sociological accounts – of 'false consciousness' – will of necessity be evaluative; and these evaluations are likely to be in terms of the ideological use of cultural resources by dominant vested interest groups to retain and spread their power and privileges. In his *The Possibility of Naturalism*, Bhaskar (1989: 63) writes:

> if ... one is in possession of a theory which explains why false consciousness is necessary, then one can pass immediately, without the addition of any extraneous value judgements, to a negative evaluation of the object (generative structure, system of social relations or whatever) that makes that consciousness necessary (and, ceteris paribus, to a positive evaluation of action rationally directed at the removal of the causes of false consciousness).

This muddies the waters for Hume and those of his disciples inclined to positivistic sociology and to a doctrinal stance on is/ought.

Bhaskar has more to say on is/ought. It is not just a matter of exposing false consciousness. Consider the wage-form in capitalist societies. The nature of this wage-form cannot be laid bare – that is, be truthfully accounted for – in the absence of a critique of capitalism as a system of class exploitation. Why is this? Creaven (2007: 17) explains:

> a scientific diagnosis is simultaneously a political-ethical critique, if, as Marx believes, the wage-form is a mechanism of alienation and exploitation. And, if this is so, specifying the nature of 'what is' (capitalism as a system of class exploitation) logically entails a specification of 'what ought' (an alternative social system in which class exploitation is abolished). This is simply unavoidable, since capitalism is not a force of nature, is not governed by natural necessity, and so is not beyond rational criticism or the powers of human agency to ameliorate or abolish.

In a nutshell, certain propositions in sociology, if true, deliver moral obligations 'by force of logical necessity'.

Sociology *must* be critical, at least in some of its studies (it is always possible to sidestep engagement, as we shall see in the field of health inequalities). To diagnose an 'is' that is detrimental to human self-knowledge or self-emancipation, 'and which is an unneeded determination of human unenlightenment and unfreedom', Creaven (2007: 18) adds:

> is necessarily to specify an 'ought' (a new state of affairs that replaces these unneeded determinations with needed ones). In other words, descriptive and analytic accuracy in social science is necessarily

supportive of evaluative judgements about the rights and wrongs of social and cultural forms.

To criticise the wage-form is to criticise an institution that delivers acquiescence to class exploitation by disseminating the erroneous belief that wages are commensurate to the real value of the commodities that wage-labourers produce. And, Creaven (2007: 18) again:

> insofar as such a diagnosis undermines the ideology of a 'fair day's work for a fair day's pay', it may contribute to proletarian struggles for abolition of the wage system.

Humans' historically generated needs and interests, namely, those that underwrite a person's physical and psychological well-being, do not simply reduce to 'wants' or 'desires'. This is because, inasmuch as social relations are capable of sustaining a level of economic output sufficient to improve 'the life chance of the entire community', it is acceptable to regard the continuing frustration of these by vested interest groups as a denial of *real* needs and interests. Creaven (2007: 19) once more:

> such constraints on human freedom would be socially and materially 'unneeded', because they are not determined by natural fetters (e.g. insufficiency of resources). Rather, they are determined by social structures and social practices that are organized in ways which preserve the power and privilege of superordinate classes or elites at the expense of the life-chances of subordinate groups or classes.

There is an argument here that such social practices are not only *morally* wrong, but *objectively* so. To continue in this vein, it is the task of a 'critical' social theory to undermine their ideological justifications and to spell out ways of achieving change. Moreover, the social struggles of the 'oppressed and exploited' *against* such structures and their beneficiaries are morally right: they are 'objectively, ethico-political "right action"'.

Explaining is a theoretical endeavour

There has long been a tendency among positivists then: (a) to regard explanation as something that emerges from data analyses oriented to prediction (as is implicit in crude, multivariate analyses that too often reduce to 'significance hunting'; and (b) to see this whole process as value-neutral. But what of theory? Theory always informs sociological practice, even when its practitioners are in denial. It guides sampling and data collection and processing as well as analysis in positivist studies. Its guidance can be overt or covert. It is overt when an explicit attempt is made to spell out and to call to account or 'test' a particular theory. It is covert when investigators are content to see what turns up. Moreover, to choose one theory to test is to neglect others; and 'what turns up' in a study is in part determined by the research design, regardless of whether it hinges on a secondary analysis of an extant data set or on ethnographic fieldwork in a particular setting.

In the next chapter I discuss in detail seven key theoretical paradigms or 'clusters' that have informed sociological examinations of health and health care, namely, structural-functionalism, interactionism, phenomenology and ethnomethodology, social constructionism, postmodernism, conflict and critical theory, feminist and post-colonial and disability theory. It will suffice here to offer a few preliminary pointers. First, to reiterate, theory intrudes into any study, like it or not. Second, it is important that sociologists face up to and are reflexive about theory's omnipresence. Third, it is possible to compare and evaluate theories and, to borrow Popper's term, to determine their respective degrees of 'verisimilitude'.

Theory in sociology can be pitched at micro-, meso- or macro-levels. Micro-sociology concentrates on our mundane everyday behaviour, much of which is rule-governed beyond our reflexivity or suspicion. Meso-sociology, which Merton (1968) famously called 'middle-range theory', collates and bridges the shores of our daily decision-making and broader and deeper social structures. Macro-sociology addresses just those social structures that, often unawares, nudge or shove us into behaviours for or against our interests. The relevance of all three branches of sociology for health and health care is obvious.

What is perhaps less obvious is their interdependency. It is in this sense that Bhaskar's concept of *totality* will later be introduced. For now, it is enough to note that no micro-sociological theory of what presents as highly individualised decision-making can be considered comprehensive in the absence of either a meso-sociological theory of why individuals in this same set of circumstances take different decisions or a macro-sociological theory of those social and cultural structures that set the broad parameters within which all such decisions are taken. For example, a micro-theory of smoking would be incomplete without both a meso-theory of addiction and a macro-theory of the marketing policies of transnational tobacco companies and their relations with governments.

There is a qualification to add. I shall maintain that sociology is not reducible to psychology, biology, biochemistry, genetics, physics and so on (any more than the latter are, as Comte boldly insisted, reducible to sociology). Nevertheless, it is axiomatic that psychologists, biologists and others have plenty of important things to say and theories to advance about phenomena like smoking. *Sociology never wraps up the phenomena it targets.* This is so not only because it deals with social structures, relations and processes rather than, say, individual cognition or affect, neuronal networks or the programming of cells, but also because of unpredictable contingency and the very real and causal role of human agency. So while this book is a discourse on sociology and the social, it will have sooner or later to say more about *interdisciplinarity.*

Sociology's necessary dip beneath-the-surface

This final sub-section is a reminder that the true of objects of study of sociology, and indeed all the other natural, behavioural or social *sciences* mentioned in passing in the previous paragraph, lie beneath-the-surface of the worlds we inhabit. They are inaccessible to the senses and it is their effects that indirectly alert us to their existence. We cannot *see* the causal mechanisms of class or gender any more than we can *see* gravity. This casts an important light on the first half of this chapter. Citing the pioneering and exciting endeavours of early epidemiogists, it was possible to document changes in the patterning of diseases leading to death and to show that these were related to 'social factors' like material and social standing and gender. It remains, however, to specify the social mechanisms that exercise some degree of causal responsibility for such associations.

If poverty, absolute or relative, is positively associated with premature demise, *why is this*? How do we get from material and social deprivation to terminal bodily harm? For macro-sociologists, what are the causes of 'material and social deprivation'? Is material and social deprivation, *together with its genesis*, best captured *sociologically* by the concept of social class? If so, which of the numerous competing concepts? And how do relations of gender – and ethnicity and ageing to cite just two further examples – 'complicate' the picture?

How, in short, does sociology maximise its potential to satisfy social – whilst fuelling interdisciplinary and more comprehensive – explanations of health inequalities? Enough has been said in this chapter to trigger the meta-constructive theory that is proffered in subsequent chapters. Moreover, there is a lot more to the sociology of health, illness and medicine than health inequalities.

Summarizing so far

In this first chapter, I have hinted at an agenda for a credible sociology of health and health care. It has been more negative than positive, highlighting problems to be solved rather than anticipating solutions. The opening paragraphs demonstrated change over time in the human lifespan. While this change seems incontrovertible, its causes remain contestable and contested. It seems that the Neolithic revolution and the transitions to stable agricultural states and industrialism were key moments; but the empirical support for such judgements raises matters of deeper and more lasting concern. As we shall see, it is not just a matter of *why* these changes occurred when they did, and with the consequences they had. Other questions arise. For example, are we misled in our interpretations of previous eras by the conceptual frameworks – lay and expert – into which we have ourselves been socialised into imposing the present on the past? There is an issue of hermeneutics here: can we faithfully recapture the past via the present? And if so, how, and at what risk?

Enough has hopefully been said to render questionable allegedly 'neutral' positivistic research. While epidemiology and public health are arguably (and understandably) prediction-led, sociology is oriented to explanation. Sociology can – indeed, has to – offer a compelling, finite, incomplete but nevertheless non-reducible explanation of phenomena like changes in mortality rates and health inequalities. Whence and whither poverty and deprivation in financial capitalism? We shall see too that health inequality offers but one focus for the sociology of health and health care. There are many other foci: how people come to define themselves as healthy or ill; what they do about it if they consider themselves ill; how definitions of health, illness and disease are influenced by ideology as well as by popular culture and expert systems; what options are available (self-care, folk healing, professional biomedicine); and so on. The second chapter casts sociological light on some of these issues via a critical explication of the dominant perspectives that underpin sociology's contributions.

2   Perspectives in health sociology

Sociology is a composite discipline. It was founded out of and survives as a broad church. There have been a number of histories of its emergence and consolidation, some theoretically driven (Gerhard, 1989), others more focused on its institutional settlement. Cockerham (2000) offers a brief account that helpfully spans the two. He dates the origins of medical sociology between 1897 and 1955. It was a paper by Henderson in the *New England Journal of Medicine* in 1935 that serendipitously sparked the interest of Harvard student Talcott Parsons. Prior to the publication in 1951 of Parsons's monumental *The Social System*, which examined the role of medicine in macro-level social systems, the embryonic sociology of medicine had been strictly oriented to practical issues of policy, treatment and care (sociology *in* rather than *of* medicine).

The years 1956–1970 marked for Cockerham medical sociology's 'golden age'. American scholars like Merton, Becker, Goffman and others strode confidently either in or avoiding Parsons' footsteps. As we shall see below, new varieties of conflict theory, as well as symbolic interactionism, dramaturgy and labelling theory, emerged to make their impact on studies of health. It was an age that culminated in 1970 in Freidson's remarkable work of synthesis, *Profession of Medicine*, a work that stands alongside Parsons' *The Social System* as a catalyst for sociologies of health and health care. This was the period too in which pioneering textbooks saw the light of day and the discipline spread out from the USA to Britain, Germany and elsewhere.

For Cockerham, the era from 1970 to 1989 revealed the discipline in its maturity. It had established its independence from medicine and well recognised domains of interest and expertise had developed. There was a choice of textbooks and specialised journals. In Britain, sociologists emerged from a long period of gestation *in* medicine to become sociologists *of* medicine and began to develop home grown expertise across specific areas of enquiry. The principal domains of focus were: social and health inequalities; doctor-patient encounters and interaction; lay beliefs; qualitative studies of coping with illness, especially long-term illness; and feminist investigations of reproductive health.

Prudently, Cockerham is more reticent on the period post-1989 and opts not to characterise it. In my own brief discussion, I identified a number of tensions that have carried over to the present, and these help provide context for the analysis that follows (Scambler, 2006). I suggested, first, that the limitations and flaws of the (masculine, white, colonial) sociologies of North America, Europe and Australasia have been exposed in the latest accelerated burst of high-tech, high-speed 'globalization' (of which more later) and can no longer be denied. This represents a serious challenge to construct a convincing *global sociology* (see Bhambra, 2015).

Second, I referred to the growing rationalization or 'McDonaldisation' of much of sociology (Ritzer, 2001). To adapt Ritzer's phrasing, the sheer irrationality of what presents as a rational system – assessing practitioners via measures of productivity and devotion to their institutions – proffers another challenge to sociologists. It is a thesis that can be over-stated, yet it remains a threat to our autonomy and independence of thought and practice.

Intimately related to these processes of McDonaldisation, third, is what I cast as the increasing neoliberal and state direction of Britain's universities during financial capitalism. This is apparent in the ideological insistence (i) that university intakes be expanded to accommodate nearly half the country's young people; (ii) that students be prepared for the workforce, via the transmission of transferable skills for example; (iii) that commissioned research be applied and 'useful'; (iv) that universities search for commercial partners to make good any shortfall in state funding; and (v) that due consideration be given to a growing role for the private sector in higher education. The basic tension here is between universities' traditional educative and newly acquired economic functions.

Fourth, I drew attention to what I called the 'postmodernization of culture' that has attended financial capitalism. Sociologists have characterised and evaluated this cultural shift in a number of ways. Modern, universalizing *grand* narratives, some have argued, have given way to a postmodern landscape of multiple 'relativized' *petit* narratives, and they see this as a positive change: they have discerned a liberating cultural turn. Others, and I lined up with them, have seen neo-conservatism in fancy dress. It is, after all, difficult to mount a rationally compelling critique of the status quo in a pick-and-mix hybrid culture.

These tensions continue to inform and play on the practices of sociologists interested in health and health care, as will become increasingly apparent through this text. I will argue strongly that we must move towards a global sociology, resist the McDonaldisation and neoliberalization of our universities and contest the postmodernization of culture; and this stance will find many an echo in the critical expositions of schools of sociological thought that follow.

The principal task now is to interrogate a number of core perspectives or schools of thought that have characterised medical or health sociology since

its inception. These are: structural-functionalism, interactionism, phenomenology and ethnomethodology, social constructionism, post-structuralism
and postmodernism, conflict and critical theory, feminist and post-colonial
theory and, a taster, critical realism. Of course, there are others, and these
will be referred to as the argument unfolds. To stress a point made earlier,
faithfulness to authors, while important, is less so than is the relevance of
their theories for the argument of this volume. Many of the sociologists cited
here are major figures, but they are best regarded for present purposes as
catalysts: while there is little merit in jackdaw-like appropriation, there is
much potential in theoretical synthesis. I draw in part here on earlier expositions and critiques (Scambler, 2002). 'Neither either nor or' is my motto.
Each of the seven perspectives will be discussed in light of four principal
queries:

1   What are the core tenets or propositions?
2   What are its strengths and weaknesses?
3   What aspects of, or topics in, the sociology of health and health care
    does it best illuminate?
4   How might its strengths feed into the kind of sociology to be outlined
    and commended in this book?

Structural-functionalism

The main protagonist for structural-functionalism in the USA was Talcott
Parsons, who set out his stall defiantly against the positivists. In an early book,
he stressed that this was because positivism denied the *purposeful* nature
of human action (Parsons, 1937). Humans, he argued, are simultaneously
'goal-oriented' and constrained. Despite the extraordinary breadth and depth
of his writings, he is remembered mostly, however, for his analysis of society
as a 'constraining' social system. Sympathetic biographer Gerhardt (2002: ix)
writes: 'although he aimed vigorously to account for the dynamics of meaning
orientation in the increasingly pluralistic modern society, he was accused of
mechanistic systems thinking fitting a hermeneutic Brave New World'.

In his classic – it is tempting to say 'discipline-defining' – *The Social
System*, Parsons (1951) sought to show that social systems are bound by
'value patterns', without which actors' behaviour would be directionless.
Value patterns, in turn, are structured by 'pattern variables'. Pattern variables denote those universal dichotomies that represent the basic choices that
underpin social interaction. These are the dichotomies:

*   *Universalism versus particularism*: actors relate to others according to
    general criteria or criteria unique to the individual concerned;
*   *Performance versus quality*: actors relate to others on the basis of criteria
    of performance or achievement or criteria of some form of endowment
    or ascription;

- *Specificity versus diffuseness*: actors relate to others for specific, restricted purposes or in a general holistic way;
- *Affective neutrality versus affectivity*: actors relate to others in a detached and instrumental manner or with the engagement of feelings and emotions.

Modernity, Parsons reasoned, has experienced a shift towards universalism, performance, specificity and affective neutrality.

On the one hand, the concept of pattern variables reflects the voluntaristic dimension in Parsons's thinking. The notion of 'functional prerequisites', on the other hand, seeks to capture the way people's relations to and interaction with others are embedded in and constrained by social systems. Social systems can only exist, in fact, if four functional prerequisites are met. These are:

- *Adaptation* (A) to the external or natural environment;
- *Goal-attainment* (G) or the mobilization of resources to meet relevant needs;
- *Integration* (I) or the accomplishment of regulation and coordination for coherence and stability;
- *Latency* or *pattern-maintenance* (L) or the provision of means to sustain actors' motivational energy.

Parsons calls this the AGIL-schema. Social systems that develop institutions capable of more efficiently satisfying all four AGIL functions gain an evolutionary advantage over other 'rival' systems.

In modernity, the argument runs, the macro-level social system of the nation state can be divided into four subsystems:

- *Economic subsystem*: concerned with *adaptation*;
- *Polity*: concerned with *goal-attainment*;
- *Social community*: concerned with integration;
- *Cultural subsystem*: concerned with *latency* or *pattern-maintenance*.

The AGIL-scheme and the pattern variables are linked at this point. For example, the economic subsystem, where adaptation is the functional prerequisite, is characterised by universalism, performance, specificity and affective neutrality. The social community, where integration is the functional prerequisite, is characterised by particularism, quality, diffuseness and affectivity.

Nor was Parsons yet done with this Germanic, Hegelian and, in his view, largely Weberian theoretical edifice. With reference to evolutionary change and modernity, he wrote of *differentiation, adaptive upgrading, inclusion* and *value generalization*. Baert (1998: 62) pulls a number of threads together:

first, with time, a process of 'differentiation' occurs in that different functions are fulfilled by subsystems within the social system ... Second, with differentiation goes the notion of 'adaptive upgrading'. This means that each differentiated subsystem has more adaptive capacity compared to the non-differentiated system out of which it emerged. Third, modern societies tend to rely upon a new system of integration. Process differentiation implies a more urgent need for special skills. This can only be accommodated by moving from a status based on 'ascription' to a status on the basis of 'achievement'. This implies the 'inclusion' of previously excluded groups. Fourth, a differentiated society needs to deploy a value system that incorporates and regulates the different subsystems. This is made possible through 'value generalization': the values are pitched at a higher level in order to direct activities and functions in various subsystems.

For Parsons, the evolution or emergence of the modern profession represented a significant breach with the past. In fact, his pattern variables were progeny of his study of professions. After the manner of Durkheim, he did not see the professions primarily as self-interested economic actors. The role of the physician, he reasoned, epitomised the modern leaning towards universalism, performance, specificity and affective neutrality. Moreover, this is functional for the relationship between physician and patient. Just as there is a discernible physician role, so was born in modernity a 'sick-role mechanism'. Health, Parsons (1951: 38) argued, 'is intimately involved in the functional prerequisites of the social system'. Too much ill or poor health is dysfunctional because it inhibits the effective performance of social roles.

Parsons maintains that there is a 'psychic element' or 'motivatedness' to illness, which leads him to define illness as a form of social *deviance*. It is a point that often goes missing from standard textbook accounts of the sick-role. Exposure to risk, even in instances of accidents and infections, often has a motivational component. Gerhardt (1987, 1989) discerns a crucial 'dual model structure' here. On the one hand, illness implies a ('negative-achievement') 'incapacity' to fulfil ordinary role responsibilities, the sick role being a 'niche in the system' to provide for recovery and rehabilitation. But on the other hand, the Parsonian accent on 'deviance', deriving from psychoanalysis, focuses on the ('positive-achievement') motivational forces at play, discerning an 'unconscious psychotherapy' incorporated in medical treatment.

As Turner (1995) demonstrates, and as should already be apparent, there is much more to Parsons of interest to medical sociologists than the concept of the sick role. He highlights his work on the non-profit ethos of the professions, on the influence of structure and culture on health and on the relationship between religion, death and the 'gift of life'. As I see it, the strength of Parsonian structural-functionalism lies in its exposure of the structural and cultural shaping of our lives, or more specifically those of Americans half a century ago. He addresses those enduring *beneath-the-surface* social forces positioning and moulding – but never entirely determining – who we are and how we act. I shall argue later that this aspect of his work was wrongly neglected through and after the 1960s, lost amongst the plethora of critiques of structural-functionalism.

There were weaknesses too of course. First, there is an issue about how Parsons's theoretical frame and propositions might be appraised empirically. How might Lawson's demi-regs add or subtract from their plausibility? They seem to hover worryingly close to Popper's non-falsifiable/pseudo-science trap. Second, it can reasonably be argued that Parsons omits, and maybe rules out of court, any proper analysis of conflict or disequilibrium. This is likely a function of his early preoccupation with social order. Boundary maintenance and internal integration came to trump dissent and fissure. Third, it is not readily apparent how Parsons's four functional prerequisites for any social system – that is, adaptation, goal-attainment, integration and latency/pattern-maintenance – *actually* secure the maintenance and survival of the system.

C Wright Mills (1963) famously lambasted systematic or abstracted empiricism at one end of the spectrum and grand theory at the other. Parsons might be judged to succeed or fail as a grand theorist. But there is more to his work than that. Notwithstanding his early motivation, agency did indeed go missing. Since his seminal outputs, however, it has typically been structure and culture rather than agency that have all but disappeared from view. First one of Dawe's (1970) 'two sociologies', then the other! If Parsons has relatively little of lasting value to feed our understanding of the *lifeworld*, his analyses of the *system* are more durable. The system, which operates beneath-the-surface and behind-our-backs, I shall maintain, has been neglected by medical sociologists, not least with respect to the mal-distribution of health and life expectancy documented in the previous chapter. The structuring of culture and agency insinuates itself into the life-worlds. To paraphrase Stevie Smith, a tiny minority surf social structures while the overwhelming majority risk drowning.

Interactionism

Interactionism in general, and 'symbolic' interactionism in particular, emerged as a lively and combative rival to structural-functionalism in the USA. It was agent- rather than structure- and micro- rather than macro-oriented. It too departed from positivism but headed off in a different direction to structural-functionalism. Its focus was on *understanding*, deriving from Dilthey via Weber's 'vertstehen', rather than causal *explanation*. A key figure was George Herbert Mead, although there were precursors. It was the Thomas partners, for example, who introduced the concept of the 'definition of the situation'. If people define their situations as real, they argued, then they are real in their consequences. And it was Cooley who pioneered the notion of 'the looking-glass self'. We form ourselves by looking in the mirror, and it is 'others' who constitute our mirror. We respond to what we see, re-evaluating our sense of who we are, our self-images, when we see the unexpected (see Ritzer, 2003).

Mead's *Mind, Self and Society*, published in 1934, was based on lecture notes. The self, he argued, must be a social self. Baert (1998) has distinguished between what he calls 'interactionist' and 'symbolic' dimensions to this social self. The interactionist dimension refers to people's capacity to adopt the attitude of other individuals and of the 'generalized other', while the symbolic dimension refers to the dependency of the social self on the sharing of symbols (incorporating the full gamut of extra-linguistic media). Another distinction has acquired a significance in accounts of Mead's work that it perhaps lacked in his lectures, that between the 'I' and the 'me'. The former stands for the acting, creative aspect of the self, while the latter represents the object of the 'I': the 'I' can only be observed, recalled or recounted as the 'me'.

Blumer (1969) built on the foundations laid by Mead. Individuals, he insisted, have social selves and possess a capacity for 'self-interaction' (a notion revisited later in the writings of Margaret Archer). Picking up on Parsons' theme of social order, however, Blumer departed from Mead to maintain that social order is reliant on people's recurrent use of congruent schemes of interpretation. Meanings are not 'given'; rather, they vary in line with people's projects: 'the actor selects, checks, suspends, regroups, and transforms the meanings in the light of the situation in which he is placed and the direction of his action' (Blumer, 1969: 5). 'Joint action' is dependent on (shared) attributions of meaning.

Now to consider Goffman, Blumer's graduate student but a friend rather than disciple of symbolic interactionism. He was a one-off theorist. He followed Blumer in eschewing 'system imperatives', but he scrupulously avoided spelling out a 'systematic' alternative theoretical framework. 'Co-presence' was his overriding theme (Gouldner, 1970). His forte was the study of rule-governed yet improvised 'performances' in face-to-face encounters. He analysed front-stage performances (e.g. when waiters served meals to their clients) and back- or off-stage performances (as they interacted with kitchen staff).

As far as medical sociology is concerned, it is his studies of asylums (Goffman, 1968a) and stigma (Goffman, 1968b) that have proved most influential. His latter account features later in this volume. Goffman was especially prescient on the routine everyday dealings of the 'discredited' (possessors of visible marks of unacceptable difference whose challenge is to manage the impressions others have of them) and the 'discreditable' (possessors of invisible marks of unacceptable difference whose challenge is to manage the information others have about them). For present purposes, however, it is Goffman's (1969) seminal *Presentation of Self in Everyday Life* that assumes the most significance. This book focuses on the structure of interaction. To expose the rules that regulate social interaction, Goffman argued, is to reveal its structure. The structure of face-to-face interaction in the lifeworld stabilises the social order. People conduct themselves in their everyday lives much as actors perform according to scripts. A number of 'ground rules' specify the means available to them to realise their goals; these provide normative regulation. One ground rule has to do with the 'maintenance of face'; this requires individuals, like actors on a stage, to present and sustain consistently positive images of the self and to acknowledge this same process in those with whom they interact. This is accomplished by acting 'lines': participants in interaction typically act to prevent lines from being discredited, thus avoiding loss of face for *all* those involved. Social life is predictable to the extent to which those who interact arrive at a working definition of the situation.

Definitions of the situation can, as Goffman recognised, reflect the distribution of power. In psychiatric units, for example, an individual's performed self can and often is challenged by others positing a rival definition. The self, in the gendered language of the time, 'is not a property of the person to whom it is attributed, but dwells rather in the pattern of social control that is exerted in connection with the person by himself and those around him' (Goffman, 1961: 168). The self, in short, is the product of an institutional nexus of performances, although rarely in the extreme form found in total institutions like in-patient psychiatric units.

Social order is maintained not only by rule-following but by rule-breaking. Echoing Durkheim, Goffman maintained that rule-breaking (or 'remedial interchanges') is pervasive. This is because social interaction is structured primarily to allow individuals the chance to 'adjust' while pursuing their personal goals with the minimum of fuss. Such rule-breaking, typically exercised through 'accounts', 'apologies' or 'requests', gets the traffic moving again (Goffman, 1971). It can and often is felicitous to overlook individuals' rule-breaking rather than to challenge them (unpunished 'deviance') (Scambler, 2009).

What some find missing from Goffman's dramaturgical sociology is any explicit acknowledgement of the external and constraining nature of Durkheimian 'social facts'. What of those meso- and macro-structures like class, gender, ethnicity and so on that provide the plots around which scripts and actor improvisations occur? In Parsons's terminology, what allowance is made for system-based influences on how people define their situations and act on these definitions? Consider again Parsons's notion of the sick role. Goffman's dramaturgy is self-evidently salient to our understanding of what Freidson (1970) called people's 'lay referral systems' and to how doctors and people who become patients interact, but it skates over the medical profession's social control 'functions'. Doctors police work attendance by controlling access to the sick role. *This is the system at work.* Although the system is comprised of people's interactions, or performances, the plot is encrypted. Doctors are no more reflexive about or signatories to their social control functions than are their patients.

In other words, while it might be that interactionists, extending to the likes of Goffman, successfully pointed an accusing finger at the structural-functionalist privileging of system over lifeworld, the baby too often disappeared with the bathwater. It will be argued here that a credible sociology of health and its distribution in national, regional and local communities requires quantitative and qualitative input at each of macro-, meso- and micro-levels. Structural-functionalist analyses of systems are qualified but cannot be displaced by interactionist analyses of the lifeworld.

Phenomenology and ethnomethodology

Schutz (1970), in his seminal *The Phenomenology of the Social World*, drew on the work of the phenomenologist Husserl in an attempt to breathe new life into a revised Weberian project. Husserl had sought to found an objective and rigorous 'new science' by solving the epistemological problems bequeathed to him by Hume's empiricism on the one hand and Descartes's rationalism on the other. Schutz was no devotee of Husserl's resultant transcendental phenomenology; but lessons were learned. I would place him a little closer to the Husserlian project to travel via radical doubt to 'the' indubitable foundations for knowledge than to the contemporary propensity to use phenomenology and the subjective as synonyms. Social reality was for him:

> the sum total of objects and occurrences within the social cultural world as experienced by the commonsense thinking of men living their daily lives ... It is the world of cultural objects and social institutions into which we are all born, within which we have to find our bearings, and with which we have to come to terms. From the outset we, the actors on the social scene, experience the world we live in as a world both of nature and of culture, not as a private but an intersubjective one, that is, as a world common to all of us, either actually given or potentially accessible to everyone; and this involves intercommunication and language.
>
> (Schutz, 1962: 53)

So social reality is for Schutz intersubjective. It follows that we share schemes of meaning. The interpretations we jointly make in our everyday lives derive from a shared or common 'stock of knowledge'. While this is in part personal and idiosyncratic, it is also inherited rather than invented afresh by each generation. Furthermore, 'our involvement in the flow of action and our use of the stock of knowledge is, in the natural attitude, one predominantly directed towards practical ends' (Anderson et al., 1986: 91). A person's stock of knowledge consists of 'typifications' that are taken-for-granted unless or until revealed as such by phenomenological reductions of the kind commended by Husserl. These typifications are organised according to a dynamic or system of *relevances* determined by a person's ever-changing interests.

The lifeworld comprises a number of social dimensions, each possessing a distinctive spatiotemporal structure. First among these is that of face-to-face relations and interactions, or the 'pure' We-relation. In this dimension, people participate in each other's conscious life, resulting in a 'synchronisation of two interior streams of consciousness' (Schutz, 1964: 26). The next dimension embraces the world of contemporaries and involves: people 'whom I informally encounter face-to-face'; people 'whom I have never met but may soon meet'; people 'of whose existence I am aware as reference points for typical social functions' (e.g. post office employees processing my mail); as well as 'a variety of collective social realities (e.g. government agencies) which exist and affect my life, but with whom I may have no direct contact' (Bernstein, 1976: 149). While face-to-face interaction is constituted principally by a 'Thou-orientation', a relation in the non-concrete social dimension of contemporaries is constituted mainly by a 'They-orientation'. Both, however, share a time zone in which others are either directly encountered or can be encountered. This does not apply to two other dimensions that Schutz spends less time analyzing, those of *predecessors* and *successors*.

Another of Schutz's signal concepts is that of 'multiple realities'. He contends that within clearly demarcated forms of social life (extending beyond everyday life to encompass fiction, science, art and so on), within 'finite' provinces of meaning, 'the systems of relevancies invoked and the stocks of knowledge available enable us to bestow the character of 'factuality' in different ways' (Anderson et al., 1986: 93). Sociologists have yet to grasp, he thought, that the subjectivity found in the lifeworld needs to be made available under the 'theoretical attitude'. This can be articulated, and developed, as follows:

> Sociologists are 'not' concerned with the experiences and meanings of actual individuals, but rather with 'typical actors' with 'typical motives' who pursue 'typical goals' via 'typical courses of action': that is, with 'second-order typifications' (or typifications of our everyday or first-order typifications). Schutz arrives at three postulates for social scientists. The first is that of logical consistency. The second is that of subjective interpretations: action must be taken as meaningful for social actors. The third is that of explanatory adequacy: social scientists cannot attribute to 'actors in the theory' anything other than common-sense theories.
>
> (Scambler, 2002: 21; and see Anderson et al., 1986)

There is a clear sense here of the ways in which Schutz, drawing on selected motifs in the philosophy of Husserl, impressively extended and deepened the pioneering work of Weber and his neo-Kantian discipleship. The principle innovator and spokesperson for ethnomethodology, Harold Garfinkel, was indebted to Schutz, as he was to the symbolic interactionists and, less obviously perhaps, to Parsons (his Ph.D. supervisor, who gifted him the problem of social order). But Garfinkel's ethnomethodology had a distinctive focus. In Ritzer's (2003: 154) words, ethnomethodology is 'the study of ordinary members of society in the everyday situations in which they find themselves and the ways in which they use commonsense knowledge, procedures, and considerations to gain an understanding of, navigate in, and act on those situations'.

Sociologists should not treat actors like 'cultural dopes', at the mercy of prevailing social structures. What Durkheim defined as external and constraining 'social facts', Garfinkel re-defined as the 'accomplishments of members'. Ethnomethodology, in other words, is focused on the organization of ordinary, mundane social life. He wrote of the *reflexivity of accounts* to refer to the fact that people constantly make sense of their surroundings and that 'these sense-making practices are constitutive of that which they are describing' (Baert, 1998: 85). Echoing Wittgenstein (1958), he argued that people know the 'rules' only in that they are skillful in acting in accordance with them. Our knowledge in mundane day-to-day affairs is tacit and practical rather than discursive or theoretical; it is 'seen-but-unnoticed'. The related theme of *indexicality* recognises, after Wittgenstein again, that the meaning of objects and practices depends on the context in which they arise.

Garfinkel (1967) practiced the ethically dubious methods he termed 'breaching experiments'. In order to expose and lay bare our rule-following – to settle on one example – he got his students to return to their parental homes and act as if they were lodgers (e.g. thanking their parents formally for services like preparing meals). Unsurprisingly, deep emotions were aroused. By such acts of defiance, he reasoned, rules his students might not have been able to articulate would stand out more starkly. But he recognised too that rule-breaking often constitutes a form of deviance for self and for others.

In the 1950s, Garfinkel had met a person named Agnes, who presented unambiguously as a woman. But Garfinkel discovered that Agnes had not always presented this way: she had been a 'boy' until the age of 16 and was at the time he met her trying to persuade surgeons to remove her male genitalia and create a vagina. Ritzer (2003: 159) takes up the story. Sensing 'something was awry' at the age of 16, Agnes ran away from home and began to dress as a girl:

> She soon discovered that dressing like a woman was not enough; she has to 'learn to act' like (to pass as) a woman if she was to be accepted as one. She did learn the accepted practices and as a result came to be defined, and to define herself, as a woman. Garfinkel was interested in the passing practices that allowed Agnes to function like a woman in society. The more general point here is that we are not simply born men or women; we all also learn and routinely use the common place

practices that allow us to pass as men or women. Only in learning these practices do we come to be, in a sociological sense, a man or a woman.

With the savvy of hindsight, there is something very prescient in these observations.

For Gerhardt (1989), phenomenological and ethnomethodological perspectives alike issue in a sense of illness as 'trouble'. With reference to therapy, a clinical paradigm is evoked. Garfinkel accents the practical as opposed to the theoretical thrust of the clinical encounter, defining it as an 'artful contextual accomplishment'. Weiland (1975) builds on this insight to argue that although clinical pursuits like medicine rely on the natural and social sciences, at its core medical work is the situational *use* of this knowledge in ever-changing, if routinised, circumstances.

Schutz and Garfinkel invited sociologists to think through and deepen their grip on how actors define and renew themselves through processes of ongoing accomplishment. They picked up on and developed themes rehearsed in various forms of interactionism. What might be said at this juncture of their contributions? They certainly add more to our understanding of the 'symbolic' than the 'political-strategic order' (Baert, 1998: 88). They show how actors deploy stocks of knowledge to reproduce and re-stabilise social order in complex if mundane ways; but they are no more forthcoming than Parsons on intentional, transformative change at the structural level. Power is the elephant in the room. Like the interactionists, they lend themselves to the sociology of the lifeworld rather than the system.

Some of Garfinkel's successors made play with the notion that only when sociologists have comprehensively come to terms with the minutiae of everyday encounters can they move on to tackle the so-called 'big questions': micro-sociology necessarily precedes and provides the base for macro-sociology. A few might still maintain this, but I will argue later that micro, meso- and macro-sociology are intertwined, and none stands alone or is foundational for the others.

Have phenomenological and ethnomethodological perspectives nevertheless fed usefully into medical sociology? It is clear that they have. The work of Schutz in particular has filtered into and informed a plethora of agency-based investigations. Ethnomethodological studies of doctor-patient encounters, extending to the 'meaning-in-use' of concepts like 'diagnosis', 'prognosis', 'therapeutics', 'prescribing' and so on, have thrown the dynamism, negotiation and spontaneity of interaction into sharp relief. How medical expertise and 'patienthood' are accomplished in dialogue is an important query for sociology.

Referring back to the previous chapter, there are questions about the choice of 'featured' subject-matter, as well as about the 'taken-for-granted' lying behind the concepts used to frame it. Why was the lens turned on the changing expectation of life at birth in the UK? And why were positivist data used even as positivism was under severe and critical interrogation?

Ethnomethodologists have forced sociologists to reflect on what they do, indeed on what 'doing sociology' is. This insistence on operational reflexivity will be confronted later.

Social constructionism

Social constructionism is a broad church. At one ('weak') end of its spectrum are those who remind us that all concepts are social and that we neglect this at our peril; at the other ('strong') end are an altogether tougher breed who limit 'knowledges' and engagement to and by time and place. Strong constructionism, as we shall see, is a step too far for many sociologists.

Berger and Luckmann (1967) are often cast as progenitors of social constructionism in their *The Social Construction of Reality*. Influenced by Schutz, they sought to combine accounts of objective structures with those of actors' agency. Their orientation, unsurprisingly, tended to the lifeworld rather than to the system. Their starting point was the stocks of knowledge that constitute people's background (cultural) assumptions about the worlds they inhabit. These give them a world – a symbolic order – that they cannot readily circumvent or turn their backs on.

In the wake of Berger and Luckmann's classic text, a significant division opened up between those who followed them in retaining the structure-agency distinction and those – strong or radical constructionists – who came to conflate structure and agency. This division crystallised into that between realists and relativists. While the realists held that there exist 'external' natural and social worlds or realities that in some way or other simultaneously enable and constrain our claims to knowledge about them, the relativists denied that there is or can be any rational basis for deciding between alternative 'conceptualizations' of reality. The relativists, in short, reduced *ontology* (what exists) to *epistemology* (what we can be said to know about what exists). Bhaskar calls this the 'epistemic fallacy' and, as we shall see, its 'exposure' was at the very heart of his emerging philosophy of critical realism.

Within medical sociology in the UK, there was an interesting and revealing exchange between Nicolson and McLaughlin (1987, 1988), who ventured a constructionist account of the different and contradictory frames implicit in vascular versus immunological theories of multiple sclerosis (MS), and Bury (1986, 1987), who was wary of constructionism per se (see McDonnell, 2013). The former contended that immunological theory prevails over vascular theory in relation to MS because of the degree of cognitive fit between its model and the clinical expertise involved in the management of the disease, plus the prevailing pharmaceutical and other orthodoxies of the day. Knowledge, it might be said, follows power. This seems unobjectionable enough.

For Bury, social constructionism is a seductive and slippery slope to relativism. If scientific knowledge is relative because it is socially constructed, then sociological accounts of scientific knowledge are no less so. This is a special case of the thesis that relativism is self-refuting: any argument for relativism must itself be relative. Surely, Bury insists, we *can* and *do* engage with scientists and physicians on the basis of a common understanding that, for example, power relations exercise a real and independent impact on health that is nevertheless open to challenge and remediation. Nicolson and McLaughlin counter that versions of constructionism like theirs are realist in the ontological sense that they neither deny the existence of power relations or of health versus disease, nor dismiss the objects of scientific and medical knowledge as mere artefacts. They rather argue that 'knowledge may be regarded not as a unique representation or mirror of external reality, but as an instrument by which we may operate with that reality' (Nicolson & McLaughlin, 1988: 251). For such 'constructionist realists':

> the explanatory power of constructionism demonstrates that the contrasting perspectives and evaluations of medical knowledge are underdetermined by the properties of an external physical reality, while over determined by social processes.
>
> (McDonnel, 2013: 118)

There is no gainsaying the heterogeneity of forms of social constructionism. Strong versions, much influenced by Foucault (of which more later), tend to suffer from the excessive enthusiasm of advocates so offended by biological determinism that they end up substituting social determinism. Some weak versions stretch beyond the trivial truth that all concepts are social to feed into credible sociological theories of health, illness and medicine. Olafsdottir (2013) presents an overview. She heralds the contributions of social constructionism to our understanding of the cultural meanings of illness; notions of normality and abnormality; people's 'contextualized' responses to illness; and the emergence and parameters of medical knowledge. She goes on to cite the power of cross-national comparisons in relation to social constructionism. But she sees weaknesses as well as strengths in its assembly of stances. It is not enough, she insists, merely to show that the world is socially constructed. Why is this salient? It is one thing, to take her own example, to document processes of 'medicalisation', quite another to link such processes to health inequalities and outcomes. Plus, she warns us again, while social constructionism provides a corrective to biological essentialism, it should not lead us into a 'similarly narrow social essentialism' (Olafsdottir, 2013: 53).

So does social constructionism offer a credible paradigm for sociological enquiry? Or do more acceptable 'weak' positions lead inexorably, even logically, to less acceptable 'strong' positions? Was Bury right to be wary? I certainly share his concerns. What is of value in social constructionism has been probed and deepened by its advocates, namely, its focus on cultural shifts and their sequelae. If simply asserting that all concepts are social and therefore susceptible to amendment and revision fails to impress, then demonstrating the contextualizing and anchoring of concepts – like health, illness, disease and medicine – in power relations and the like is important and helpful. It is part and parcel of doing sociology well, for example, that the as yet largely unexamined concepts introduced in the previous chapter are subjected to investigation in their own right. The lessons of social constructionism must be taken on board even as, I shall contend, the ambitions of its more radical adherent are reigned in.

Post-structuralism and postmodernism

If social constructionism is a lively and occasionally squabbling kinship network, then post-structuralism and postmodernism comprise a hyperactive, post-squabbling, post-kinship network; or at least they did until recently. Post-structuralism and postmodernism have often been used as synonyms. Others demand their differentiation. To search for clarity across discourses is to search for a needle in a haystack. Foucault, on whom I shall concentrate here, has been labelled a post-structuralist *and* a postmodernist. Post-structuralism denotes a position emergent from and influenced by ('objectivist') structural accounts of society and social change, *but one that represents some sort of moving on* (Bourdieu has been cited). Postmodernism, on the other hand, is in my view, a bin into which all sorts of garbage have been rightly assigned; *but it has left its mark*. So how is it to be defined and assessed?

In a previous text, I took on the thankless task of explicating and critiquing what was at the time described as the 'postmodern turn' (Scambler, 2002). It was then and is now apposite to come to terms with the idea of 'postmodernity' as well as that of postmodernism. I quoted Eagleton at some length (1996: vii–viii). Postmodernity, he averred, is:

> suspicious of classical notions of truth, reason and objectivity, of the idea of universal progress or emancipation, of single frameworks, grand narratives or ultimate grounds of explanation. Against these Enlightenment norms, it sees the world as contingent, ungrounded, diverse, unstable, indeterminate, a set of disunifying cultures or interpretations which breed a degree of skepticism about the objectivity of truth, history and norms, the giveness of natures and the coherence of identities. This way of seeing, as some would say, has real material conditions: it springs from an historical shift in the West to a new form of capitalism – to the ephemoral, decentralized world of technology, consumerism and the culture industry, in which the service, finance and information industries triumph over traditional manufacture, and classical class politics yield ground to a diffuse range of 'identity politics' ... Postmodernism ... is (a form of culture which) reflects something of this epochal change, in a depthless, decentred, ungrounded, self-reflexive,

playful, derivative, eclectic, pluralistic art which blurs the boundaries between 'high' and 'low' culture, as well as between art and everyday experience. How dominant or pervasive this culture is – whether it goes all the way down, or figures as one particular region within contemporary life is a matter of argument.

My own general characterization of how its proponents see 'the postmodern' is summarised in Table 2.1, adapted from Scambler (2002: 32). My explication here will be brief. Under the rubric of 'material', a case can be made for an acceleration of processes of globalization in both economic and cultural realms. Economically, such processes are typically articulated in terms of the abstraction of capital and the ascendency of financial capital. Giddens (1990) stressed also the distanciation or separation of time and space, which has paved the way for the 'disembedding' of social relations from their local contexts, chiefly through symbolic tokens like money and expert systems like repositories of technical knowledge. Closely associated with these changes is the putative decline of the nation state, especially of national structures of political and economic regulation. This, in turn, is linked with what many proclaim to be a terminal crisis in welfare statism. Power, it is frequently said, is more diffuse than hitherto. In Foucauldian terminology, surveillance, technologies of the self and governmentality have supplanted former loci of domination like class and state (Foucault, 1977).

Table 2.1 Dimensions and Elements of the Postmodern

Material
Globalization and the ascendancy of financial capital
Decline of the nation-state and of national regulation
Crises in postwar welfare states
Diffusion of power
Emergence of societies based on consumption not production
De-standardization of work
Class decomposition and de-alignment
Displacement of class by consumer identities

Cultural-aesthetic
Postmodernism and the problematizing of reality
De-differentiation of value-spheres and de-privileging of science
Tendencies to nihilism and fundamentalism
Glocalisation in relation to culture

Rationality
Expiry of universal reason
Termination of flawed Enlightenment meta-narratives
Celebration of fragmentation and dissensus
Intellectuals as interpreters not legislators
New reflexivity

Methodological
Polyphony and dialogue
De-centring of author's authority

Consumer society, the argument runs, has displaced producer society in what has become a post-industrial formation. 'Fordist' or assembly-line modes of production have ceded ground to de-standardised or segmented work patterns orientated to consumerism. There has been class decomposition or dealignment, which is linked to a new emphasis on gender and ethnicity as dimensions of stratification. Identity-formation is now pivotal, privileging notions not only of identity but of difference. Class identities have lost their salience, the switch being to consumer identities ('you are who you choose to buy to be').

What of the cultural-aesthetic elements of the postmodern? 'Postmodernism' emerged as an aesthetic movement in the 1960s and is associated with

> the effacement of the boundary between art and everyday life; the collapse of the hierarchical distinction between high and mass/popular culture; a stylistic promiscuity favouring eclecticism and the mixing of codes; parody, pastiche, irony, playfulness and the celebration of the surface 'depthlessness' of culture; the decline of the originality/genius of the artistic producer; and the assumption that art can only be repetition.
> (Featherstone, 1991: 7–8)

Some commentators understandably labelled this 'second-wave modernism', but postmodernism has a more radical edge: whereas modernism made *representing reality* problematic, postmodernism makes *reality* problematic. Moreover, postmodernism reaches beyond art to penetrate culture as a whole. And furthermore, it renders permeable not merely the boundary between art and everyday life but those between science, morality and art; in other words, it de-privileges science. It has been said that this opens the door both to nihilism and to fundamentalism as people covet the security of absolutes in a relativistic culture. The tendency towards the global, finally, is associated with a tendency towards the local (and a kind of re-tribalisation), leading to the coining of the word 'glocalisation' (Roberston, 1992).

The rational elements of the postmodern coalesce into five principal theses. The first heralds and celebrates the implosion of all forms of universal reason. Nor is it necessary, Rorty (1989) insists, that the default option is some form of relativism. It follows from the demise of universal reason, however, that the progressive and often teleological, not to mention masculine, white and colonialist, meta-narrative of the eighteenth-century European Enlightenment be finally abandoned. Hence the Kantian 'project of modernity' – to deploy reason to travel steadily towards the good society and life – dies too. We inhabit a post-meta-narrative world. As Lyotard (1984) expressed it, we are faced with unconstrained choices of petit narratives. We must rejoice at fragmentation and the triumph of dissensus over consensus. Implicit in these changes is a newly fashioned role for the intellectual: s/he has become an 'interpreter' instead of the 'legislator' for modernity (Bauman, 1987) (check out the panellists on the BBC's 'Question Time', a current affairs discussion programme). Finally, the postmodern turn has thrown up a new reflexivity. The world, Giddens (1990: 38) suggests, is now 'intrinsically sociological': social practices are incessantly examined and reformed in light of incoming information about those very practices.

Methodologically, the postmodern has been associated with pluralism. Polyphony, dialogue and eclectic mixes of methods are commended. Ethnography, for example, no longer represents, but 'evokes'. As a natural concomitant, the authority of the author is diminished and rival voices, otherwise sidelined or suppressed, are distinguishable from the background noise of modernity.

Post-structuralism and/or postmodernism had a considerable impact on medical sociology, although they now seem to have had their day in the sun (Cockerham, 2013). Foucault, frequently cited as a post-structuralist *and* a postmodernist, has been the major catalyst. Foucault was by no means a pioneer, however, in stepping back from biomedicine and acknowledging the social construction of notions of health, illness, disease and medicine. Freidson (1970), in critiquing Parsons, drew on a mix of interactionism and conflict theory (see below) to argue that professions of medicine not only prognosticate on, and legitimate or deny, people's 'acting sick', but actually create the social possibilities for them to do so. Freidson left a 'biological base', however, beyond the reach of sociology. What Foucault did was *commandeer this biological base*.

Foucault moved much further across the spectrum of social constructionism. What we recognise as diseases, he argued, are rather fabrications of powerful discourses. Foucault (1977: 138) stripped the subject of its creativity and analysed it 'as a complex and variable function of discourse'. At the root of his corpus was the notion of the *episteme*, which 'constitutes' subjects during specific historical periods. In *The Birth of the Clinic*, Foucault (1989) traces the emergence during the nineteenth century of a *clinical gaze*, that is, a new way of conceptualizing the patient's body (the prerequisite for a novel form of medical practice). The result, 'scientific medicine', was not the product of a reasoned progression in understanding; it represented a displacement of one incommensurable 'anatomical atlas' by another (Armstrong, 1987). Moreover, this shift was part and parcel of more general macro-social processes of change.

As European capitalism went through its neophyte stages, it was accompanied by population expansion and urbanization. Extant forms of social control – largely coercive and exemplary – faded and were replaced by others, notably surveillance of self or 'self-monitoring'. Bentham's 'panopticon' was the model for and epitomy of self-monitoring. Imprisonment was the starting point: a circular building around a central tower, Bentham maintained, would mean prisoners would feel they were under constant observation even if they were not, and as a consequence, they would start policing their own behaviour. This panoptic principle, Foucault argued, had spread to inform the whole of society. He referred to *disciplinary society*, a society under-written by surveillance of self. Annandale (1998: 36) notes how the diffusion of panoptic power through the whole of society 'is evidenced in the growth of psychiatry and its urge to confess; in the growth of preventive medicine which relies on the internalization of powerful discourses of healthy diets and fitness regimes; and in self-help techniques (such as weight-control groups)'. These 'humanistic discourses', Annandale adds, are far from benign: they actually represent a new and ultimately more repressive kind of power over modern individuals. Foucault (1980: 155) puts it succinctly. There is now:

> no need for arms, physical violence, material constraints. Just a gaze. An inspecting gaze, a gaze which each individual under its weight will end by interiorizing to the point that he is his own overseer, each individual thus exercising this surveillance over, and against, himself.

What a cost-effective mechanism of social control, Foucault exclaims. And this was before today's epidemics of CCTV!

As Petersen (2012) has shown, Foucault's influence on the sociology of health and health care has been particularly significant. In the UK, for example, Armstrong (1995) soon announced the emergence of 'surveillance medicine'. Moreover, Foucault's resonance is fading more slowly than that of other post-structuralists and postmodernists. *Medicine's contribution to social control no longer assumes the form of exclusion or repression, but rather of inclusion and normalization.* His pioneering analyses of the relativizing of bodies are proven catalysts for putative postmodern sociologies of the body (see Scambler, 2002). Foucault offers – as it were, on behalf of strong constructionists – an abiding and challenging series of reflections. But he has rightly been critiqued, and compellingly. I would emphasise two criticisms. The first is a repetition of the earlier contention that (strong constructionist) forms of relativism are self-refuting. Foucault, as Habermas (1989) insists, is in 'performative contradiction': to be convincing he must assume what he has explicitly rejected, namely, the force of the rationally compelling, or better, argument. While there is merit to Foucauldian examinations of 'regimes of truth', whatever the results its progenitors still need 'to reserve their own take on the truth apart from whatever regimes they examine' (Porpora, 2015: 203); and there's the trap they cannot escape from.

My second criticism is related. It is that while Foucault excelled on *how* power slips and slides into and infuses social institutions, his relativism required him to neglect *why*. If he leavened Marxist and Frankfurt School notions of largely class-based 'dominance', he also, as theorists so often do, lost the baby with the bathwater. As we shall see, there exist abiding structural, cultural and agential uses and abuses of power that do not reduce to prevailing knowledges.

I dislike the term postmodernity, which to me speaks of too deep a rupture. I prefer to write of (a) a new phase of capitalism, which I call financial capitalism (of which much more later) and (b) a companion cultural shift, which is often said to herald the advent of postmodern culture but which here I shall term consumer culture. There is no doubt that this consumer culture has many of the characteristics identified by post-structuralists and postmodernists. What can and must be taken from the writings of social constructionists and their sometimes hot-headed and unruly post-structuralist and postmodernist offspring is an appreciation of the power implicit in discourse and those of power's tributaries that lap gently and sometimes unseen far away from primary riverbeds. But, there exist, I shall affirm later, material realities – and other constituents of the 'real' – that are *extra-discursive*.

Conflict and critical theory

Any account of conflict theory must start by interrogating Marx. He insisted that men act on the external world through 'labour', changing both it and themselves in the process. Labour is a social process. And different types of society are discernible, each one characterised by a discrete set of needs met by a discrete means of organizing labour. Marx rejected all extant political economies theorizing society as 'aggregates of individuals'.

Capital, he argued, is 'one element in a definite social relationship of production corresponding to a particular historical formation and is only manifested in things, such as the spinning jenny' (Keat & Urry, 1975: 99). *All* social phenomena are relational: the notion of wage-labour, for example, cannot be grasped without reference to that of capital. There are no natural or general laws of economic life that are independent of given historical structures. Thus, economic 'laws' address things that are social rather than natural and need to be seen as specific to a particular 'mode of production'.

Most political economies, Marx emphasised, trade only in surface appearances: they do not dip beneath-the-surface. It is 'commodity fetishism' in capitalist societies that leads to this divergence between (surface) appearance and (beneath-the-surface) reality. Commodities are objects produced that have simultaneously a *use-value* (that is, a usefulness to their consumers) and an *exchange-value*. But objects are produced for their exchange-value. Moreover, people come to see the exchange-value of any particular commodity not as a product of labour, but as a 'naturally given fixed property of the commodity' (Keat & Urry, 1975: 100). Commodities assume 'thing-like' relations with each other. *What is social comes to be viewed as natural.* Commodity fetishism, in short, disguises real social relations of production: they do not appear for what they are. Marx condemns any positivistic social science stuck at this fetishistic level of appearances as false and misleading.

It is the commodification of labour power that was for Marx the distinguishing feature of capitalism. Wage-labourers may have formal freedom, but in the absence of any alternative means of subsistence they effectively become 'wage-slaves'. Moreover, what might be considered 'value-added' is entirely down to labour power. Whether *in fact* labour power comprises a process of value-adding depends on capital's capacity to control workers in the labour process: productivity is critical. Control and productivity are essential for the 'exploitative' appropriation of the *surplus value* created by labour. Jessop (1998: 26) summarises:

> the struggle between capital and labour to increase productivity (by extending the working day, intensifying effort during this time, or boosting output through cost-effective labour-saving techniques) is the fundamental basis of the economic class struggle in capitalism. Class struggle is not simply about relative shares of the capitalist cake. It is rooted in the organization of 'production' itself (the labour process) and not just in 'market relations' (including struggles over wages) or 'distribution' (including distribution through the state). It concerns not only the accumulation of money as capital but also the overall reproduction of capital's domination of wage-labour in the economy and wider society.

Marx certainly deployed a notion of 'functional interdependence' in relation to the capitalist mode of production, though he would have had no truck with the kind of structural-functionalist explanation later espoused by Parsons. There are after all functional needs to be satisfied in all modes of production. But Marx emphasised the relations of domination that have characterised all forms of society (excepting primitive communism). These are based on the contradiction between the dominant and the dominated.

Two of capitalism's functional needs come together in this contradiction. First is the need for satisfying the 'capitalist function': buying labour power and directing its uses in capitalist enterprises. And second is the need to satisfy the 'labour function': selling labour power and producing exchange-value for the capitalist. Only if these functions are met can capitalism sustain and reproduce itself, *yet they are in contradiction.* Capitalists pursue their profits through accumulation, but this can only be achieved at the expense of those who provide the labour power. Over time, Marx (1933: 39) wrote:

> if ... the income of the worker increases with the rapid growth of capital, there is at the same time a widening of the social chasm that divides the worker from the capitalist, an increase in the power of capital over labour, a greater dependence of labour on capital.

This structural contradiction sits at the core of capitalism in all its guises.

Marx's 'method of abstraction' has a special significance to arguments I develop in the next chapter. In his *Grundrisse* (Marx, 1973), he contended that one cannot adequately analyze a given population in terms of properties like its urban-rural divide or occupational structure. Rather, one must pose questions of its classes. The analysis then shifts from the concrete to 'abstract general principles'. The scientific method, for Marx, involves deploying abstract general principles to reconstitute the concrete as a complex combination of many determinations, a 'unity of the diverse'. A given population is not seen abstractly but as determined by the 'rich totality of many determinations and relations' (Marx, 1973: 100; Scambler, 2002).

Marx is neither the only classical conflict theorist nor the sole role model or inspiration for contemporary practitioners. By the same token, neo-Marxism is a heterogeneous category. I have opted here to focus on the Frankfurt School in general and Habermas in particular because of their significance for later chapters. Horkheimer and Adorno's (1972) *Dialectic of Enlightenment*, written during the Second World War and published in 1947, set the tone for early work within the School. In the shadow of the Holocaust, it conveys a sense of decay and gloom. Habermas was to distance himself from his mentors' equation between rationality and what Weber called *Zweckrationalitat* or 'instrumental rationality'. Instrumental rationality refers to the rationality that governs the choice of means to given – often material – ends. Habermas came to contrast this with 'communicative rationality', which refers to the process of reflecting on our background assumptions about the world and 'bringing our basic norms to the fore, to be questioned and negotiated' (Braaten, 1991: 12). Instrumental rationality takes these background assumptions for granted. Furthermore, Habermas contended, instrumental rationality cannot account for 'cultural evolution', or even for economic and administrative systems, which are just too complex (Scambler, 2001a).

There is space here only to summarise two core theses in Habermas's wide-ranging analyses. I shall focus on: (a) his defence of universal reason and (b) his portrayal of modernity's de-coupling of system and lifeworld and its ramifications (Habermas, 1984, 1987). His search for universal reason yielded a formal or procedural concept of rationality. It was rooted in the subject-subject relations of communicative action. Habermas's telling intuition was that people's use of language implies a common endeavour to attain consensus in a context in which all participants are free to contribute and have equal opportunities to do so. Language use, in short, presupposes a commitment to an 'ideal speech situation' in which discourse can realise its full potential. It does not follow that an ideal speech situation can easily be attained, but it does mean that communicative action, although always occurring in a particular cultural context, rests also on an *ahistorical factor*. Brand (1990: 11–12) summarises well. This ahistorical factor, he writes:

> is found in the claim for the validity of the reasons which induce people to take their particular share in communicative action. In such claims no historical limitation is recognized since they are based on the (implicit) view that their validity should be accepted by anyone capable of judgement who is free to use it, whether in the past, present or future. The idea of rationally motivated shared understanding – and rational

motivation implies the total lack of compulsion or manipulation – is built into the very reproduction of social life, or so Habermas claims. The symbolic reproduction of society is based on the 'counterfactual' ideal of the 'ideal speech situation', which is characterized by 'communicative symmetry' and a compulsion-free consensus.

(see also Scambler, 1996)

One primary strand of commentary on Habermas's work insists that he was above all else committed to combining two principal and rival approaches to social theory. The first analyses society as a meaningful whole for its participants (*verstehen* theory), while the second analyses society as a system stabilised behind the backs of its participants (system theory) (Sitton, 1996: 168). In his two-volume *Theory of Communicative Action*, this gave rise to Habermas's celebrated distinction between the *lifeworld,* based on social integration, and the *system,* based on system integration. The lifeworld resists easy defining: it cannot be 'known' since it is the vehicle of all knowing. It is not something that individuals can step outside, although elements can and are occasionally called into doubt or 'thematised', that is, made the subject of disputation as participants attempt to re-establish their definition of the situation, a prerequisite for successful cooperation.

The system denotes material rather than symbolic reproduction and is characterised not by communicative action but by (instrumental or) 'strategic action'. There is more than a hint of Parsonian sociology here. Societal differentiation, Habermas argues, has produced four subsystems: the economy, the state and the private and public spheres of the lifeworld. Moreover, modernity has also delivered a fundamental 'de-coupling' between the economy and the state, comprising the system, and the private and public spheres, constituting the lifeworld. These subsystems are interdependent: each is specialised in terms of what it produces but is dependent on the others for what it does not produce. The economy produces 'money', the state 'power', the private sphere 'commitment' and the public sphere 'influence'. These products or media are traded between subsystems. For example,

the economy relies on the state to establish such legal institutions as private property and contract, on the public lifeworld to influence consumption patterns, and on the private lifeworld to provide a committed labour force, and itself sends money into each other subsystem.

(Crook et al., 1992: 28)

We have witnessed a progressive de-coupling of system and lifeworld. The media, and hence subsystems, of the former have come to dominate the latter. In a manner that has echoes of Weber (on rationalization) as well as Marx (on commodification), the lifeworld has become 'colonised'. In other words, it becomes increasingly state-administered, or 'juridified', and commercialised. Possibilities for communicative action in the lifeworld become attenuated as social participation becomes hyper-rationalised in terms of immediate returns. Participants encounter each other as legal entities and parties to contracts rather than as acting subjects. System rationalization has outstripped the rationalization of the lifeworld; expressed differently, western rationalization has been 'selective'.

Habermas distances himself from the 'iron cage' pessimism of Weber. He charges Weber with regarding the West's rapid system rationalization and lifeworld colonization as inexorable and inevitable, while it was in fact contingent. Weber conflated the *dynamic* and the *logic* of development. The latter, Habermas contends, allows for further rationalization of the lifeworld – that is, for an extension of the scope of communicative action and communicative rationality – and, it follows, for lifeworld 'de-colonization', notably through a reconstitution of its public sphere.

So why did system rationalization outpace and trump lifeworld rationalization? How did the colonization of the lifeworld occur? Much was down to the welfare state that emerged to fill in the 'functional gaps' or deficits of capitalism occasioned by the economic disequilibria of crisis-ridden growth due, for example, to business cycles and infrastructural under-investment. The welfare state also emerged because of the potential for class struggle over distribution. This potential was blocked by corporatist devices resulting in wage scales set through bargaining mediated by the state and by the direct state provision of use-values like health and social care. In this way,

> the social antagonism bred by private disposition over the means of producing social wealth increasingly loses its structure-forming power for the lifeworld of social groups, although it does remain constitutive for the structure of the economic system.
>
> (Habermas, 1987: 348)

With the steady postwar rise in standard of living, together with other state-sponsored protections from system imperatives, 'conflicts over distribution also lose their explosive power' (Habermas, 1987: 349–350). The rising standard of living and protective policies of the welfare state reduced the salience of the role of employee and enhanced that of the consumer. The class structuration of the lifeworld, together with the proletariat, slipped out of view (Sitton, 1996).

It is a moot point whether, or to what extent, Habermas has retained his enthusiasm for Marx. It is however possible both to query his fidelity *and* to learn from his synthesis of prior schools of sociological thought. So what might provisionally be concluded from this selective précis of conflict theory? In the case of Marx only, too often infants and young children as well as babies have been lost with the bathwater. His analysis of societal development and differentiation through changing modes and relations of production still resonates. If his analysis is now dated, as indeed it must be and is, it is often misunderstood or liable to ideological distortion. The theoretical input in subsequent chapters draws on Marx's laying of foundations.

As for Habermas, and notwithstanding his progressive distancing from the writings of Marx, he provides a useful conceptual framework. I shall argue that his version of critical theory lacks a plausible ontology but has a worthwhile epistemological return. I shall draw explicitly on his theory of communicative action and his analysis of system/lifeworld de-coupling; but I shall also introduce others of his theoretical-cum-substantive contributions, most conspicuously on 'legitimation crises' and, an unhappy phrase, the 'feudalization' of the public sphere.

The scripts of Marx and Habermas are alike pertinent to the sociology of health, illness and medicine (Scambler, 2001b, 2002). Consider the data on the maldistribution of morbidity and mortality presented in the previous chapter. Representing a theory-bound but constipated and non-reflexive neo-positivism, these data sit in an odd vacuum. But Navarro in particular has consistently and over a long period demonstrated not only *how* the theories of Marx and neo-Marxists (maybe *just* including critical theorists like Habermas) can cast explanatory light on the production and reproduction of health inequalities but *why* they have been overlooked. Grouping people by their occupational status, incomes or characteristics of their employment falls short, Marx and critical theorists insist; sociologists must do better than passively adjust to or accommodate epidemiological research. They must have their own agenda.

Feminist, post-colonial and disability theory

Feminist, post-colonial and disability theory are indebted to social and sociological research even as they reach beyond and challenge it. There is a pivotal distinction to be made between sociologies of gender, race or ethnicity and disability, which have long masculine, white and 'able-ist' ancestries, and feminist, post-colonial and disability theory. The paragraphs that follow focus on some of the ways the latter confront, contest and distance themselves from the former. There continues to be a lively debate about as to whether sociology can 're-connect', and I address this later.

It has become commonplace to discern three, or more polemically four, *waves* of feminism, each associated with a distinctive theoretical orientation. While this modern, western division into waves 'overlooks' those pre-modern, non-western women's movements that are being painstakingly resurrected by feminist historians, it provides a useful frame. Definitions and characterizations are nevertheless hard to come by. The first wave is typically linked to the late nineteenth century/early twentieth century fight for equal opportunities in general and suffrage in particular. One 'herstory' celebrates its birth at the Seneca Falls Convention in 1848 and Elizabeth Cady Stanton's subsequent declaration culminating in a political strategy for change. Britain was not in the vanguard of progressive change: the vote for women aged 21 or more was won only in 1928 (15 years after Emily Davison's death at Epsom's Derby). This and other pioneering engagements by women necessarily required a 'liberal' re-examination of the differences between men and women.

The second wave was more explicitly theoretical. Emerging around the 1960s, it was the sister of a plethora of other minority, anti-Vietnam and civil rights movements. Equality of rights was a signature. Its theories reflected a fusion of neo-Marxism and psychoanalysis. The subjugation of women was associated with wide-ranging critiques of patriarchy, capitalism, normative heterosexuality and women's roles and scripts as wives and mothers. Sex and gender were clearly differentiated, the former being *biological* and the latter a *social construct* variable by time and place. While the first wave was largely championed by middle-class, white and cisgender ('cis' being a neologism referring to those whose gender and sexual identities map clearly onto one another), protagonists of the second wave drew in women of colour and from developing nations in pursuit of sisterhood and solidarity. Many proclaimed that 'the personal is political' and that gender, ethnic and class oppression are interrelated. Others insisted on women-only spaces and argued that women were more humane, collaborative, inclusive and holistic in problem-solving than their male counterparts.

Feminism's third wave had its origins in the mid-1990s and was informed by post-colonial and postmodern thinking. The general effect was to destabilise many constructs that had been taken for granted. Garfinkel might have called it a natural breeching experiment: concepts like 'universal womanhood', 'body', 'gender', 'sexuality' and 'heteronormativity' were interrogated and rendered suspect. 'Grrls', 'cybergrrls' and 'netgrrls' eschewed victimization and took over feminine beauty for themselves *as subjects*, not as objects, of a sexist patriarchy. Sexist culture was subverted via terms like 'slut' and 'bitch'. The third wave was characterised by irony. Ambiguity was celebrated: gender boundaries could be crossed, most conspicuously in cyberspace. Grrl feminism became global, multicultural and postcategorization. Difference was positively cast and reality framed as performance and contingency. In many respects, feminism's third wave belonged 'in the academy'.

The parameters of a putative, or embryonic, fourth wave are less transparent. It is represented mostly by the activities of young feminists outside of the academy at once rediscovering and refashioning earlier theories and aspirations. Solidary initiatives against sexual abuse, rape, violence against women, unequal pay, slut-shaming, conformance to body-type and lack of representation in government and boardrooms have become part of mainstream cultural issues. The fourth wave can perhaps best be defined via the notion of 'intersectionality', pioneered by women of colour. This recognises that women's suppression can only be adequately understood in the context of the 'marginalization of others'. The oppression of women and sexism co-exist with classism, racism, ageism, able-ism and so on. Inclusion is prioritised. Past feminisms are not merely reincarnated; rather, fourth wave feminism is invested afresh in the millennials.

Post-colonialism also stands against most orthodox sociologies. Its departure was marked by the publication of Said's (1995) *Orientalism* in the late 1970s. He and other critical literary scholars provided what Bhambra (2014) has termed the canonical hub of post-colonial studies. Since then it has retrospectively incorporated contributions from writer-activists like Fanon, Memmi and Cesaire and moved forward on to generate its own distinctive frames and narratives. In essence, post-colonialism interrogates and critiques the assumptions that underlie prevailing dominant discourses – including those deployed by sociologists – through which we make sense of the social world we dwell in. This involves some deep mining to destabilise prevailing ways of seeing. Spivak (1990) writes of 'reversing, displacing and seizing the apparatus of value-coding'.

An allied family of theorists has clustered around the concept of 'decoloniality'. These theories focus on existing forms of the 'coloniality of power' and/or the 'coloniality of being'. Maldano-Torres (2007: 263), who emphasises the latter, engages with the critical theory of Habermas amongst others. He argues that instead of writing as Habermas does of the 'unfinished project of modernity', we should proclaim the 'unfinished project of decolonisation'. In similar vein, Wynter (2003: 322) writes of 'a new principle of nonhomogeneity' consolidated around the 'Colour (cum Colonial) Line'.

Post-colonial and decolonial commentators are committed not only to exposing the taken-for-granted in conventional sociological practice, but also to showing how we might move forward. Just as feminists have sought to pick up and shake sociologies of gender and sexuality in order to construct more apposite understandings and explanations using some of the pieces, so theorists of the post-colonial have sought to disassemble and reassemble sociologies of race, ethnicity and colonialism.

Disability theorists rebelled against prevailing and ubiquitous cultural biases that distinguished between the desirable and normal 'able-bodied' and the undesirable and abnormal 'dis-abled'. Medical sociology too was a ready target. Inspired by the interactionist and dramaturgical schools mentioned earlier, sociologists focused – notably in the UK in the 1980s – on chronic or long-term illnesses and disabilities as 'personal tragedies'. They not only disrupted biographies and frequently led to stigmatization, they heralded unequivocally and irredeemably negative states and identities with which those affected had somehow to 'cope' whilst pursuing with whatever vigour left to them strategies of 'normalization'. Oliver (1990) was among the first to demand a *gestalt shift*. His 'social model of disability' stressed who was doing the labeling and why, not the miseries and challenges of being labeled. The notion of *oppression* was key.

There was some affinity between second-wave feminism and Oliver's rewriting of disability via a social model that was part and parcel of a critique of capitalism. Moreover, his model was community midwife to a reinvigorated 'disability politics'. The model soon came under attack, however, not least by fellow disability theorists and activists. If there is a singular way of characterizing this assault, then it might be through the catch-all notion of 'identity politics'. Self-identity, it was maintained, is at the heart of any worthwhile cultural change and effective disability politics. Barnes and Mercer (2003: 130) take up the story:

> However, while disabled activists were promoting a group identity culture and politics, they found themselves increasingly challenged by the transition to an identity politics that became a 'celebration of difference' ... Now the emphasis on a disabled identity was criticized for being in conflict with a truly emancipatory politics. Indeed, no limits were placed on the amount of difference or the distinct collectivities that might emerge, in terms of age, gender, 'race' and sexuality, for example, to undercut the claims of a common, disabled group identity.

Disabled identities, in short, were uncertain, fluid and liquid rather than solid.

These paragraphs on feminist, post-colonial and disability theory have only given a flavour of innovative and committed endeavour and activism. Each offered an overdue challenge to sociologists reluctant to reflect on premises taken-for-granted. I have owned up to my own sins of omission and commission in relation to the sociological study of long term or chronic illness and disability in the 1980s (Scambler, 2004; see also Thomas, 2007). It is not that all prior research is defunct (its studies continue to provide grist to sociology's mill), but rather that its limitations and lack of reflexivity and bite have been starkly exposed. Worse, it has been solicitous to or accommodated: (a) enduring social hierarchies of gender, sexuality, ethnicity, disease, disability and so on, and (b) their accompanying mindsets or 'isms'.

The question for me is whether or not sociology can adapt to these critiques and reconnect. I can understand those who think not. Bhambra (2014) has argued that so deep-seated are orthodox sociology's extant premises that the only viable option – and here she draws eloquently on post-colonial and decolonial theories – is not for one but (the title of her book) for 'connected sociologies'. This is not my preference, as I hope this volume will make clear. While I am largely accepting of the critiques of those conventional sociological epistemologies and practices targeted by feminist, post-colonial and disability theorists, I shall nevertheless argue for reconnection and a unified sociology allied to Habermas's reconstructed 'project of modernity'.

Another summary

So what point have we reached? This chapter has surveyed a selection of sociology's principal schools of thought and enquiry and appended an appreciative and/or critical comment or two. It should be clear that each school excites more than the varieties of positivism on display in the previous chapter and adds to sociology's potential even as it disqualifies itself as its sole representative. Parsons's focus on the system-like properties of our social world is as valuable as the mundane, everyday or lifeworld proclivities of Mead, Goffman or, for that matter, Schutz or Garfinkel. Syntheses can be fruitful, as Habermas demonstrates. In these summary observations I want to stress two points.

The first is that sociology cannot *and must not* be expected to wrap up our understandings and explanations of whatever phenomena are of interest to us. It is not just that happenstance is important: stuff occurs *contingently*. Nor is it merely that we have to factor in *agency*, that is, a human capacity for decision-making. These are of course salient, but so too is the need to recognise that the mechanisms that generate change exist and are simultaneously active at different levels of reality. As a convenient shorthand, I shall continue to refer to biological, psychological and social mechanisms. Although mechanisms at each of these strata are simultaneously active, they are 'non-reducible': for example, although the social is 'emergent from' the psychological, which is in turn 'emergent from' the biological, it is *not* reducible to either. Social mechanisms, I shall argue, can and must be examined *in their own right, but they can of necessity only tell part of the story*. Our DNA and personalities impact on who we are and what we do, but sociology remains a vital, intact and scientific enterprise oriented to the 'good society'.

The second point is that sociology presents in multiple guises. Burawoy (2005) delineated four sociologies: *professional, policy, critical* and, his juncture of advocacy, *public sociology*. This typology has been extended by means of two additional ideal types: *foresight* and *action* sociology (Scambler & Scambler, 2015). Foresight sociology refers to sociological work oriented to experimental 'alternative futures', for instance in terms of green technology, public housing, social mobility or participation in wellbeing. Action sociology denotes engagement beyond public sociology to insist on or compel – against the ideologies of vested interests – attention to its scientific output.

Table 2.2 alludes to the preliminary and largely socio-epidemiological consideration of health inequalities in Chapter 1. It addresses the six types of sociology via the device of sample questions that might be expected to arouse the curiosity of sociologists (see Scambler & Scambler, 2015). It will be immediately apparent that this sextet of queries covers ground beyond any territories colonised by epidemiology. A companion observation is that each and every one of the sociological theories or perspectives so skimpily introduced above might fruitfully come into play in attempts to answer them.

I end by anticipating a theme that will run throughout this volume and for which my few paragraphs on feminist, post-colonial and disability theory have a special salience. While I entirely accept that each of this trio of theory clusters has become detached from an often halting, hesitant, obdurate, paternalistic, white discipline of sociology, I shall argue strongly that sociology: (a) must remain a 'science of society'; (b) is necessarily oriented to what

Table 2.2 Six Sociologies and Six Questions on Health Inequalities

---

Professional sociology
Which social structures, relations or mechanisms are causally critical for health and longevity in which contexts and through each phase of the lifecourse?

Policy sociology
How might evidence-based research on health inequalities most effectively be translated into telling interventions?

Critical sociology
What obstacles emanating from power relations contaminate/neutralise sociology's comprehensive array of contributions to research on health inequalities and its dissemination and impact?

Public sociology
What kinds of routes and media offer the best prospects of participatory public engagement in decision making pertaining to health inequalities"

Foresight sociology
How might different types of organizational and/or institutional change deliver a more equal distribution of health and longevity?

Action sociology
How might sociologists best resist being 'rubbished', ignored or sidelined on health inequalities by those with a vested interest in a status quo conducive to their widening and deepening?

Source: Adapted from Scambler & Scambler (2015).

Habermas calls 'system decolonisation' and 'lifeworld rationalisation'; (c) must aspire to be 'global', therefore not masculine, white and Occidental; (d) must, if it is to make progress on (c), open itself up to learn from and adapt to the likes of feminist, post-colonial and disability theory; and (e) can accomplish (a) to (d). If I am right and not just cheerfully optimistic, sociology must face up to some very severe critiques and criticisms. Chapter 3 begins this process by developing philosophies and theories presented and applied by Habermas, Bhaskar, Archer and others.

Part II

3 Basic critical realism and health

Although philosophical and theoretical in many respects, it is not my intention in this text to be 'faithful' even to those – like Habermas and Bhaskar – to whom I am most indebted. The intent is to 'do sociology'. I am content to take what I want or need from predecessors and consociates. Habermas, for me contemporary sociology's creative synthesiser-in-chief, has formal-epistemological and substantive offerings. I shall make routine use of his procedural account of reason and rationalization, his framing of system and lifeworld and the former's colonization of the latter. Bhaskar, who retains a stronger Marxist pulse than Habermas, is decisive in his insistence on making up for what he calls the 'epistemic fallacy', that is, the notion that we have come to reduce 'reality' to what we can or might be said to know of it; in other words, we have collapsed ontology into epistemology. At the core of his project is the recapture of the real. He prepares and nurtures soil Habermas has left uncultivated.

Bhaskar's critical realism has been mentioned but only in passing. I make use here of both its 'basic' and 'dialectical' guises. In this chapter I concentrate on the former. It was Bhaskar's mission to rescue ontology from what he judged to be decades of scandalous neglect. Too many philosophers, he maintained, have fallen for the 'epistemic fallacy', that is, they have reduced what *is* to what we can be said to *know* about what is. In spelling out his 'realist ontology', he distinguished between three basic strata of reality, the *empirical*, the *actual* and the *real*. The empirical is the world as apprehended by experience; the actual is the world of events; and the real comprises those structures or 'generative mechanisms' that *must* exist for us to experience events in the ways that we do. The real:

> is not uniform, but is multi-layered, with lower-order structures (such as the brain and central nervous system) giving rise to higher-order structures (such as mind and consciousness). The relations between these strata are based on ontological rootedness (of higher on lower) and emergence (with higher being made possible by the causal interaction of the lower).
>
> (Creaven, 2007: 8)

Bhaskar's stratified ontology allowed him to avoid charges of: (a) reductionism, or the view that the objects of the higher sciences are ultimately reducible to those of the lower sciences; and (b) dualism, or the view that reality is composed of different and autonomous substances that interact in what Creaven calls an external and inessential way (e.g. mind and matter). He continues:

> on the one hand, reductionism is rejected because the generative mechanisms comprising a particular stratum, though generated by those of its root stratum, are nonetheless 'sui generis', a new form of complexity, with its own distinct properties and powers (such as the mind's capacity to think, which is not a property of the individual cells that compose the brain). On the other hand, dualism is rejected because stratification and emergence also mean that the relations between the objects of knowledge are not inessential or contingent, but are 'necessary', with the higher order strata only 'relatively' autonomous of their root stratum.
>
> (Creaven, 2007: 8)

There is a lot packed into this! It should already be apparent, however, that Bhaskar's ontology: (a) allows for a distinctively sociological contribution to understanding and explaining issues around health, disease, medicine and health care systems; (b) rules out any Comte-like aspirations sociologists might nurse to take control or 'wrap things up'; and (c) invites the *interdisciplinary* pursuit of ever more comprehensive understandings and explanations.

As far as epistemology, or the philosophy or theory of knowledge, is concerned, Bhaskar has an anti-empiricist and anti-positivist stance. His 'naturalism' promotes a unity of natural and social science. He acknowledges constraints on this unity, however, due to differences in methodology and what Creaven calls 'structure'. Methodologically, sociologists cannot investigate phenomena of interest to them under laboratory conditions. These phenomena exist in what Bhaskar calls an *open system*. The structural constraint is that sociology's objects of knowledge (social relations) 'are internally rather than externally related, quite unlike the relations between the socially generated natural sciences and their *non-social* objects of knowledge' (my italics) (Creaven, 2007: 9).

So what about the unity of the natural and social sciences? Their methods are certainly not identical. Yet, first, they share the same goals, namely, the pursuit of causal explanations for phenomena of interest. And second, 'it is the nature of objects that determines their cognitive possibilities *for us*', so that the form of possible science in both the social and natural domains is given by the properties (enablements and liabilities) of their respective objects of inquiry' (Creaven, 2007: 9). In other words, there can be no credible epistemology in the absence of ontology.

So, to reiterate once more, the search for natural and social scientists alike is for those real objects or mechanisms that must exist for us to experience events as we do. 'Attention', as Fleetwood (2002: 67) maintains in relation to the social sciences, 'turns away from the flux of events (constant or otherwise) and towards the *causal mechanisms, social structures, powers and relations* that govern them.' These mechanisms are 'intransitive': they exist whether or not they are detected. It is not of course possible simply to map the effects of mechanisms at the level of events and our perceptions of them. Such is the nature of an open system. This is because mechanisms act 'transfactually': once set in motion, they continue to exert an influence even if other counter-vailing mechanisms annul or prevent this influence from manifesting itself. Fleetwood cites the notion of *tendencies* employed in Marxist economics here. Thus, the mechanisms that combine to issue in the tendency of the rate of profit to decline act transfactually, that is, they are remain active even when empirically the rate of profit is rising. Their transfactuality is down to the operating of other mechanisms – such as technological advances – acting in a countervailing manner (Scambler & Scambler, 2013: 84).

Ontology for Bhaskar (1987) is not only stratified but *transformational.* What he terms his 'transformational model of social action' is intended to trump rival accounts of agents and structures. Agents, he asserts, do not create or produce structures *ab initio*, but rather *re*create, *re*produce and/ or *transform* a set of pre-existing structures. The total ensemble of struc-tures comprises/*is* society. One of Bhaskar's (1989: 129) more celebrated paragraphs reads:

> people do not create society. For it always pre-exists them and is a nec-essary condition for their activity. Rather society must be regarded as an ensemble of structures, practices and conventions which individuals reproduce and transform, but which would not exist unless they did so. Society does not exist independently of human activity (the error of rei-fication). But it is not the product of it (the error of voluntarism).

Creaven (2007: 8) argues that a 'strong account of human nature' and of the 'non-social object' is indispensable for a credible theory of structure and agency. Human nature and the non-social object denote 'an ensemble of species powers, capacities, dispositions and psycho-organic needs and inter-ests' that must exist if we are to account for the existence of human society:

> at the same time as humanity's species-being and attendant powers and capacities are transmitted 'upstream' into social interaction and socio-cultural relations (supplying the power which energizes the so-cial system, constraining and enabling socio-cultural production and reproduction, and providing a certain impetus towards the univer-sal articulation of particular kinds of cultural norms or principles), structural-cultural and agential conditioning are transmitted 'down-stream' to human persons (investing in them specific social interests and capacities, shaping unconsciously much of their psychological and spiritual makeup, and furnishing them with the cultural resources to construct personal and social identities for themselves.

It is time to show how this abstruse family of narratives might frame and open up empirical research in the health domain (see Scambler et al., 2010). I shall draw here on research on epilepsy-related quality of life (ERQOL). Epilepsy can be defined as a tendency to recurrent seizures: its aetiology often still uncertain, it is a symptom not a disease. It is disputed whether there exist 'objective' markers of ERQOL or whether ERQOL is an inherently 'subjective' notion. Obviously objective and subjective, ERQOL need not correspond: epilepsy following severe brain damage might by common consent be associated with poor objective ERQOL without translating into a poor subjective ERQOL. Geneticists, neurologists, general practitioners, clinical psychologists and health sociologists are likely to agree, however, that, to deploy an expedient shorthand, each of *biological, psychological* and *social* mechanisms can have a potent bearing on both objective and subjective ERQOL.

The causal history of ERQOL is frequently complex. For example, negative effects of epilepsy can be experienced in the absence of any salient genetic or biological structures or mechanisms, such as when epilepsy is misdiagnosed: application of the diagnostic label can in and of itself – by authoritatively foisting an unwelcome and stigmatizing social identity on a person-cum-patient – trigger psychological or social mechanisms to adverse effect. If on the other hand epilepsy is but one symptom of an underlying pathology, biological mechanisms can cancel out or override the causal potential of psychological or social mechanisms. Genetic predisposition and brain insult can also be mediated by psychological mechanisms that over time 'decide' ERQOL. The causal efficacy of psychological mechanisms like internal versus external locus of control can themselves be dependent on contexts or shaped by social mechanisms, or, for that matter, contingent happenings or agency.

The lesson here is that biological, psychological and social mechanisms can vary in their causal efficacy from individual to individual as well as by social or cultural context. Moreover, they can and often do 'interact': one genus, acting upstream or downstream, can annul or ameliorate the impact of others. Critical realism allows for this fluidity. Danemark et al. (2002: 55) elaborate:

> The objects have the powers they have by virtue of their structures, and mechanisms exist and are what they are because of this structure; this is the nature of the object. There is an internal and necessary relation between the nature of an object and its causal powers and tendencies. This can also be expressed as follows (Collier, 1994: 43): 'things have the powers they do because of their structures ... Structures cause powers to be exercised, given some input, some 'efficient cause', e.g. the match lights when you strike it'. This in turn is an example of a mechanism having generated an event. A mechanism is that which can cause something in the world to happen, and in this respect mechanisms can be of many different kinds.

At the time of writing, Bhaskar et al. (2017) have just published a more comprehensive account of the relevance of a critical realist perspective for understanding 'interdisciplinarity and well-being'.

So a mechanism operates when it is being triggered. Unlike the internal and necessary relation between objects and their causal powers, however, the relation between mechanisms and their effects is *external and contingent*. The reason? Underlying phenomena in the domain of the actual are many biological, psychological and social mechanisms that are currently active. Thus, ERQOL is a complex effect of influences emanating from an array of multi-level mechanisms, where some mechanisms can either reinforce or frustrate others. Danemark et al. (2002: 56) again:

> taken together this – that objects have powers whether exercised or not, mechanisms exist whether triggered or not and the effects of the mechanisms are contingent – means we can say that a certain object 'tends' to act or behave in a certain way.

Thus, numerous and fortuitous circumstances can play their part in determining whether a specific causal power will manifest itself or not.

To illustrate causal complexity in open systems, consider a vivid hypothetical case study presented by a previous co-author of mine, the late neurologist Anthony Hopkins (1987: 124–125):

> Consider a man with a moderate genetic disposition to seizures. Add the effects of a moderate cranial injury some two years before. Add also the effects of 'stress' at the office during the preceding month. Add also the effects of amitriptyline prescribed to help with the depression associated with this stress. If this man then has a seizure after consuming a moderate amount of alcohol the night before, what caused it – the genetic propensity, the cranial injury, the stress, the alcohol and associated metabolic changes, the disturbance of sleep associated with the depression, or the amitriptyline? *Depending upon the perspective of the world of both patient and neurologist* (emphasis added), agreement may be reached to blame just one or all of these factors, quite illogically.

ERQOL cannot be understood or explained solely in terms of *social* mechanisms (although sociology can make its own discrete and irreducible contribution). Not only do biological mechanisms typically matter, but psychological mechanisms typically mediate people's handling of biologically induced 'impairments' – as Carol Thomas (2007) calls them – in socially induced contexts. Further complications arise with unannounced contingency in human affairs and the play of human reflexivity and agency. In brief, sociology's research programmes on ERQOL only tell part of the story. And even genuinely interdisciplinary (biological + psychological + social) research programmes would not tell the whole story: the explanatory power generated would not be matched by an equivalent predictive power: people and their circumstances can and do defy science.

Basic critical realism shows a threefold return here. First, it prescribes an adequate ontology of objects, powers/mechanisms and tendencies in open systems, and does so without falling foul of the naturalist fallacy, namely, some form of reductionism Second, it demands and facilitates a move beyond the ubiquitous positivistic pursuit of statistically significant associations between variables, be they biological, psychological or social, or, more rarely, some combination of these. And finally, it calls for methodological rigour even as it denounces positivistic 'textbook' emphases on measurement via operationization and quantification using ever more advanced forms of multivariate analysis. Even Blumer might be appeased. The denunciation here is not of these positivist accessories per se, but rather of the underlying assumption that phenomena can be predicted, and therefore explained, given 'empirical' study of the 'actual', that is, without Bhaskar's 'real'. The potential for experimental closure in open systems is exaggerated.

It does not follow that extant positivistic research is redundant: it is grist to the mill of sociological endeavour, offering up 'clues' as to the nature of the real. Goldthorpe (2016) offers an argument in similar vein in his *Sociology as a Population Science*. But he departs from critical realism in that he finds no effective role for qualitative as opposed to quantitative sociology. While he allows space for retroductive inference to underlying mechanisms via quantification, he closes it down for abductive inference to such mechanisms via ethnographic or qualitative investigations.

In relation to ERQOL, more than science is at stake, however. A considerable body of research is driven by an instrumental concern to improve objective/subjective ERQOL. In an earlier piece, I ventured a frame for interventions arising out of my 'hidden distress model of epilepsy' (Scambler, 1989; Scambler et al., 2010). This model acknowledged that biological mechanisms, extending from genetics to the neuropharmacology of antiepileptic drugs, typically *matter* in relation to ERQOL, deeper understanding often mitigating epilepsy's assault on people's day-to-day lives via more effective treatment. Yet even severe biological insults 'may not' be decisive for ERQOL. Psychological mechanisms typically *condition* people's handling of epilepsy's assault, and therefore its impact on ERQOL, independently of biological severity or intractability. There is considerable scope for counselling, targeting the interface between enduring psychological states and coping styles. Yet psychological mechanisms too 'may not' be decisive for ERQOL. Social mechanisms typically provide people with *contexts*, some of which prove decisive for ERQOL. Spontaneous reactions to a witnessed seizure can be pivotal in the long as well as the short term. But social mechanisms too 'may not' be compelling for ERQOL.

My hidden distress model of epilepsy accords primary significance to 'felt stigma', referring to a sense of shame and a fear of being discriminated against on the grounds of unacceptable difference (or 'enacted stigma'). Felt stigma frequently predisposes to fearful secrecy and compromised aspiration. This led me to draw on Bourdieu to postulate an *epilepsy habitus*. This denotes an enduring, context-induced mindset, informed above all by felt stigma, which predisposes to acquiescence or passivity with regard to socially disadvantaging difference. Anticipating enacted stigma, people with epilepsy, I found, often (learn to) do to themselves what they anticipate others will inevitably do to them. An epilepsy habitus can form independently of either biological or psychological mechanisms and tendencies, although it too might lose salience for ERQOL, for example in the presence of uncompromising biological (e.g. severe brain injury) or psychological (e.g. a strong internal locus of control). Clinical and public health interventions might reasonably aim to prevent the development of an epilepsy habitus.

Revisiting health inequalities

Hopefully enough has now been said to commend basic critical realism to sociologists of health, illness and medicine, for all that the proof of the pudding remains in its eating, digestion and after effects. In the opening chapter, I detailed the evolving documentation of health inequalities in the UK and the longstanding association between reduced longevity and diminished health and poverty, disadvantage and lower socio-economic status. I argued that positivistic socio-epidemiological research oriented to prediction was appropriate for urgent public health interventions but inappropriate for a sociological project oriented to explanation. So how might critical realism underwrite a credible sociology of health inequalities? I divide what follows into four sections. In the first I address those macro-aspects of the social that have taken us phase-by-phase into what I characterise as post-1970s 'financial capitalism'. The *mal-distribution* of health, past and present, cannot be explained sociologically, I maintain, in the absence of a macro-sociology of Comte's fields of social statics and social dynamics. I draw here on various perspectives précised in Chapter 2. In the second section, I proffer a sociological theory of health inequalities for the present. In the third I apply this theory to 'reforms' to health care systems, with specific reference to England's National Health Service (NHS). Finally, I offer a provisional account of just how critical realism and the class/command dynamic are crucial for a credible sociology of health and health care in contemporary Britain.

Sociology and financial capitalism

For Marx, *contradiction* is a structural property of a system that necessarily generates dysfunctions for that system. Thus, class struggle and periodic crises are necessarily generated by capitalism but are dysfunctional for capitalist society. Such contradictions are 'internal'. Contradiction in this sense allows Marx to avoid charges of utopianism. It is not, Collier (2002: 156) writes, at the behest of a 'view from nowhere' that capitalism is resisted, 'but because capitalism has contradictions which we can see from inside it, which hurt the people inside it, and which could be resolved with the resources produced by it, but only by its abolition'.

I have over a number of years focused on the transition from post-WW2 'welfare' to post-1970 'financial' capitalism (see Table 1.1) (see Scambler & Scambler, 2013, which I draw on here). In particular, I have argued that financial capitalism is characterised above all else by a new, or shifting, dynamic between 'relations of class' (in Habermas's subsystem of the economy) and 'relations of command' (in his subsystem of the state). This revised *class/command dynamic* is for me the prime macro-sociological generative mechanism for financial capitalism. It is also, as I hope to show, the key to unlock a damagingly circumspect sociology of health inequalities.

The instability of capitalism, as Marx observed, is down to its contradictions, and these possess the potential to transmute into full-blown crises. Buechler (2008: 58–59) discerns four pertinent internal contradictions. The first is between social production and private appropriation. Production in capitalism is organised socially, requiring the coordinated input of many people; but appropriation is private and individual. Capitalism is commendably efficient at producing private commodities like televisions and iPhones but deficient at producing public goods like health care. A second contradiction is between the strategic rationality of increasingly transnational corporations and the economic 'anarchy' of the wider society. Under capitalism, there is little economic coordination or planning either for commodity or for labour markets or for core services like education, health and welfare. This is more of a threat to those in low-income households than those whose assets serve to protect them. A third contradiction involves the polarization of wealth and poverty. As capital becomes more concentrated in fewer hands, the rich become richer; and even when workers' living standards improve, those of owners of capital typically improve more rapidly. The polarization of rich and poor on a global scale is especially extreme. And fourth, capitalism produces for profit, not use. It privileges profit over need. Production for profit instead of use creates further instability by permitting the exceptional affluence of the few to coexist with the unmet needs of those less privileged.

Contradictions can transmute into economic crises, for instance in the event of over-production or under-consumption. Though such 'crisis tendencies' cannot be eliminated, they can be managed. In Buechler's (2008: 60) words, 'the dance of crisis tendencies and counterstrategies offers important insights into capitalist economies.' During liberal and into early Fordist capitalism, from 1820 to WW1, the market provided 'system integration' by coordinating the production and distribution of material goods, and 'social integration' by providing norms, values and identities that reinforced people's economic motivation. Convictions about equal opportunity, upward mobility, the work ethic and that endeavour would be recognised and rewarded were more commonplace than they were in the interwar years and thereafter. Because system and social integration were indebted to the market, liberal capitalism was highly prone to crisis. This was to change with the shift through late Fordist to welfare capitalism, dating roughly from WW1 to 1970.

Post-WW2 welfare capitalism in particular diverged markedly from its predecessor. It was corporate rather than market dominated. Transnational corporations began to monopolise production, set prices and manipulate demand, thereby nullifying any 'free' market benefits of competition, price reduction and so on. It was an era characterised too by far more state intervention, which was in part a response to liberal capitalism's failure to deliver system and social integration. The state came to underwrite core but unprofitable goods and services: maintaining the infrastructure; subsidizing education and training for workers; providing social insurance for the unemployed, people with disabilities and the retired; and addressing and mitigating the ecological by-products of capitalism. The risk of crisis was elevated in welfare capitalism. This is because it was characterised by massive state interventions to cauterise its internal contradictions and the conflicts they spawned, thereby displacing potential crises from economy to state. As Habermas (1975) noted back in the 1970s, state interventions can trigger 'crises of legitimation'.

So what of the current phase of financial capitalism? The scene has to be set. In the 1970s, the American abrogation of Bretton Woods together with the rise of the Eurodollar freed up money capital from national regulation by central banks. The international recession drew banks further into the global arena. The consequences were as follows: (a) the emergence and consolidation of transnational finance as internationalised banks established closer relations with transnational corporations, and (b) the resurgence of money capital in the major capitalist economies. Commentators wrote of processes of *financialisation*, referring not only to de-regulation and internationalization, but also to (a) a shift in the distribution of profits from productive to money capital, accompanied by an increase in the external financing of industry, and (b) a reorientation towards the financial sphere that reached into the heart of 'industrial' corporations. Carroll (2008: 55–56) writes:

> the constellation of interests atop major firms have shifted from salaried managers and bankers, towards institutional shareholders and, at certain junctures of corporate restructuring, private equity outfits.

Industrial capital has come more and more to resemble financial capital:

> as stock options align corporate management with a money-capital standpoint and as firms ... come to depend less on productive activities and more on income from financial sources.
>
> (Carroll, 2008: 56)

In the financial sector itself, Carroll continues, de-regulation has precipitated capital centralization in banks with global reach whose activities encompass both financial production and speculation in derivatives, even as institutional investors controlling capitalised deferred wages have become significant centres of allocative as well as strategic power. And on top of this exploded the global financial crisis of 2008–2009.

Unsurprisingly in light of these transformations, what I call the 'capital executive' in financial capitalism differs significantly from its predecessors (the concept as well as the terminology here is borrowed from Clement and Myles (1987). In Table 3.1 I have outlined a new classification of social class, together with a few explanatory notes. Financial capitalism's class/command dynamic is at its core, but I shall take a slightly circuitous route in showing how and why. Ironically given his doubts about the salience of class, a convenient starting point is C. Wright Mills' classic study *The Power Elite*. Since its publication in 1956, times have changed of course: the elite-versus-mass industrial society of the USA in the 1950s differs in many respects from post-industrial Britain in the second decade of the twenty-first century.

Table 3.1 New Classification of Social Class

CATEGORY (A): *Capitalist executive* (significant, largely transnational and 'detached' owners of capital)

SOCIAL CLASS I **CAPITAL MONOPOLISTS** (hard core of heavy capital-owners who are 'players') SOCIAL CLASS II **CAPITAL AUXILIARIES** (soft auxiliary core of heavy capital-owners who are non-players) SOCIAL CLASS III **CAPITAL 'SLEEPERS'** (insider higher management, light capital-owners who support players)

CATEGORY (B): *New middle class* (managers in the service of capital)

SOCIAL CLASS IV **INSIDER HIGHER MANAGERS** ('co-opted' higher/middle managers who support players) SOCIAL CLASS V **OUTSIDER HIGHER MANAGERS** (higher managers, independent of players) SOCIAL CLASS VI **MIDDLE MANAGERS** (middle managers, independent of players) (*P*) SOCIAL CLASS VII **CAPITAL ASPIRERS** ('aspirational', petit-bourgeoisie, independent of players) (*P*)

CATEGORY (C): *Old middle class* (established professionals)

SOCIAL CLASS VIII **INSIDER PROFRESSIONALS** ('co-opted', high-status professionals who support players) (*P*) SOCIAL CLASS IX **OUTSIDER PROFESSIONALS** (high-status professionals, independent of players) (*P*) SOCIAL CLASS X **SEMI-PROFESSIONALS** (semi-professionals, independent of players) (*P*)

CATEGORY (D): *Working class* (waged workers)

SOCIAL CLASS XI
INSIDER WORKERS ('co-opted', supervisory, waged workers, support players) (*P*)
SOCIAL CLASS XII
OUTSIDER WHITE-COLLAR WORKERS (non-manual waged workers, independent of players) (*P*)
SOCIAL CLASS XIII
OUTSIDER BLUE-COLLAR WORKERS (waged manual workers, independent of players) (*P*)
SOCIAL CLASS XIV
OUTSIDER SEMI/UNSKILLED WORKERS (waged semi- and unskilled manual workers, independent of players) (*P*)

CATEGORY (E): *Working class* (outside paid work)

DISPLACED WORKERS (never worked and long-term unemployed) (*P*)

Notes:
Within the capital executive there exists a hard core of heavily 'globalised' capital owners personally committed to the accumulation of capital (or material) assets. I define these as 'detached'. This fraction of the 1% constitutes the class driver for order/change, exercising its will through the offices of those in the political elite, whose members have mostly been recruited or are allied to the capital executive. The governing oligarchy's personnel are – and this is the key sociological point – surfers of a revised class structuring of British society in financial capitalism (which is, as intersectionalists remind us, also structured by gender, ethnicity and so on).

I have made a distinction between supporters and non-supporters or players. This is important because the less than 1% critically 'rely on' the co-option of others in the capital executive, new and old middle classes and even the working class. This is not a matter of elector\al or infrastructural support but of a compact of interest. These are people – from managers and accountants to lawyers and physicians to supervisors and union officials – whose cooperation with the governing oligarchy has been directly or indirectly hired or bought: they profit from the liaison.

The term 'precariat' appears (now as (p)) in parentheses. I do not accept that Standing's precariat is a class in- let alone or for- itself. But I certainly accept that there is a structural and cultural precariousness associated with financial capitalism. I here regard this as a cross-class matter placing an emboldened question mark after the security and wellbeing of most members of the new, old and working classes (90+% of the population as a whole). My employment of 'precariat' acknowledges this insecurity without making the 'error' of discovering a new class.

Sociologists should in my view be focusing far more attention on: (i) the 0.1% who comprise a cabal of globally heavy-hitting owners of capital who buy sufficient national state power to secure governance sufficient to further their agendas and interests; (ii) the 2% or so who comprise a governing oligarchy; and (iii) the maybe 7%–8% of 'supporters' and 'co-optees' (represented in each of the class categories (A) to (D)) who are critical for the viability of this governing oligarchy.

(*Continued*)

This is not to commend a focus on Savage's wealth elite, though that would be of interest. What I am arguing for here is an acknowledgement that it is the increasingly concentrated ownership and control of (largely inherited) capital that is the prime mover in financial capitalism. *This is a class issue*: a cabal within the capitalist executive buys sufficient power for its needs in the continuing absence of a crisis of government legitimation. This *class/command dynamic* is for me the principal macro-level 'generative mechanism' for financial capitalism. It delivers a governing oligarchy that, *pace* Mills, also controls, and is currently via-anti-terrorist legislation extending its control, over core social institutions of oppression and repression (from the mainstream media to MI5 and MI6 through to the armed forces and the police).

So, returning to Mills, here are a few urgent and under-researched questions for my neo-Marxist sociology of the present: (a) how are we to chart the emergence and describe the standout features of the *habitus* of those who comprise the governing oligarchy? (b) what of 'interlocking memberships' of the class-centred cabal of prime capital owners and the state's power elite – how do Mills's statistics for 1950s USA stand up for Britain in 2016? (c) how determinate and porous are the boundaries between 'tacit co-ordination' and conspiracy for the governing oligarchy? and (d) by what means is the 'higher morality' of the governing oligarchy institutionalised, and how might it be publicly and effectively contested?

There have been several mentions of Mills' text during financial capitalism. There has also been an occasional journalistic attempt to re-invigorate and apply his concepts to contemporary times (Williams, 2006). Sociologists, however, have been more ready to cite Mills than to engage with his theory of interlocking business, political and military elites, either theoretically or empirically. This was not always the case: there were several full-bloodied excursions into his domain of contention in the 1950s and '60s (Domhoff & Ballard, 1968). The power elite Mills discerned in 1950s USA comprised the corporate chieftains, the political directorate and the warlords. His choice of terminology was pointed:

> the simple Marxian view makes the big economic man the 'real' holder of power; the simple liberal view makes the big political man the chief of the power system; and there are some who would view the warlords as virtual dictators. Each of these is an oversimplified view. It is to avoid them that we use the term 'power elite' rather than, for example, 'ruling class'.

> (1956: 277)

Mills stressed the structural coincidence of elite figures' interests, as well as the overlap in their origins, education and careers that fostered a psychological affinity. Perhaps incongruously given his skepticism about the language of class, he refers to a strong class consciousness:

Nowhere in America is there as great a 'class consciousness' as among the elite: nowhere is it organized as effectively as among the power elite ...for by class consciousness, as a psychological fact, one means that the individual member of a 'class' accepts only those accepted by his circle as among those who are significant to his own image of self.

(1956: 283)

In other words, members of Mills's power elite shared a common *habitus*; that is, 'a subjective but non-individual system of internalised structures, common schemes of interpretation, conception and action' (Bourdieu, 1980: 60). Following on from this, there is a family of three concepts in Mills's analysis that are especially pertinent here.

The first of these acknowledges the *interlocking memberships* of the three domains of the power elite. It is not just that they had similar family backgrounds, schooling and Ivy League exposure, but also that there was a high rate of inter-marriage and transfer. The power elite comprised a complex, dynamic web or network of interrelations.

The second concept is *tacit co-ordination*. Mills writes:

I have tried but cannot resist highlighting this concept of 'tacit co-ordination', a sure sociological substitute for 'conspiracy'. It suits the activities of members of our current oligarchy.

(1956: 69)

His point is that members of the power elite rarely need to conspire given their *habitus*. Fight like cats and dogs though they did with their domain rivals, they retained a sharp sense of collective, inter- and intra-domain interests.

The third component of this triad is that of *small decisions*:

the power of the elite does not necessarily mean that history is not also shaped by a series of small decisions, none of which are thought out. It does not mean that a hundred small arrangements and compromises and adaptations may not be built into the ongoing policy and the living event. The idea of the power elite implies nothing about the process of decision-making as such: it is an attempt to delimit the social areas within which that process, whatever its character, goes on. It is a conception of who is involved in the process.

(1956: 21)

For all that Foucault came to neglect *who* exercised power and *why*, there is more than a hint of his subtle explication of *how* power is diffused and exercised in this statement.

Two further arguments advanced by Mills are relevant here. The first hinges on another of Mills's innovative concepts, that of a *higher immorality*. Once again quotation best serves our purpose:

> within the corporate worlds of business, war-making and politics, the private conscience is attenuated – and the higher immorality is institutionalized. It is not merely a question of a corrupt administration in corporation, army or state; it is a feature of the corporate rich, as a capitalist stratum, deeply entwined with the politics of a military state.
>
> (1956: 343)

And:

> the higher immorality, the general weakening of older values and the organization of irresponsibility have not involved any public crises; on the contrary, they have been matters of a creeping indifference and a silent hollowing out.
>
> (1956: 345)

Finally:

> a society that is in its higher circles and on its middle levels widely believed to be a network of smart rackets does not produce men of conscience with an inner moral sense; a society that is merely expedient does not produce men of conscience. A society that narrows the meaning of 'success' to the big money and in its terms condemns failure as the chief vice, raising money to the plane of absolute value, will produce the sharp operators and the shady deal. Blessed are the cynical, for only they have what it takes to succeed.
>
> (1956: 347)

The final remark on Mills anticipates Piketty (2014). Noting change over the decades leading up to the 1950s, Mills records a growing propensity for members of the USA's power elite to inherit rather than 'earn' their wealth:

> in earlier generations the main chance, usually with other people's money, was the key; in later generations the accumulation of corporate advantages, based on grandfather's and father's position, replaces the main chance.
>
> (1956: 115–116)

By the 1950s, only 9% of the very rich came 'from the bottom'; 68% came 'from the upper classes'. Possession, typically via inheritance, was already key. As so often in sociology, continuity and discontinuity battle it out. In some ways, Mills's analysis is specific to time and place; in others, it has retained its bite.

Capitalism survives but in new format and guise. I have discussed in some detail novel and continuing processes of financialisation. The following summary theses give a wider context (see Scambler, 2012a; 2012b, 2014).

Financialisation

That capitalism has entered a new phase over the last generation is not contentious. Scarcely more so is the proposition that it has undergone a form of 'financialisation'. We have witnessed a transition to what has variously been deemed high, late, reflexive, liquid, post- or second modernity; postmodernity; post-industrial or consumer society; and so on. In fact, sociologists have queued up to encapsulate the present in an apt word or phrase. The concept of financialisation, in line with the macro-theories of Giddens (1990) on 'space-time distantiation' and Castells on 'networked society', here denotes the increased speed and salience of flows of capital within and between nation-states. Billions of dollars can be shifted in milli-seconds, affording select protagonists – namely, those placing the larger bets in today's (another 'apt phrase') 'casino capitalism' – exercise an enhanced causal responsibility for others' incomes, living conditions and wellbeing. The result of such processes, I shall maintain, is a *fractured society*.

Glocalisation

The word 'glocalisation' catches financial capitalism's novel tendency to nurture global *and* local change. Inter- and intra-continental and national boundaries both count for less, hence the burgeoning literature on globalization, and for more, leading to devolution and an emphasis on localisation. Many a political elite must look outwards and inwards. This has important implications, as we shall see, for Mills's space- and time-bound elucidation of the power elite: his concepts of interlocking membership, tacit co-ordination and higher immorality require re-anchoring. As far as contemporary concepts of globalization go, it is the ubiquity of neoliberal economics that is most striking. Neoliberalism, I shall contend, constitutes an ideology at the end of/beyond ideology.

Post-ideological relativity

Financial capitalism is characterised by the surpassing of at least one core aspect of modernity, whatever terminology is deployed to describe it. As Lyotard (1972) long ago claimed, a few singular, western, Enlightenment-oriented *grand* narratives (for or against capitalism) have been displaced by a plethora of rival pick-and-mix *petit* narratives. This has left the neoliberalist status quo lacking in competition. Moreover, each and every petit narrative is now viewed as an ideology, allegedly leaving consumers free to choose their worlds and identities. Expressed in 'classical' sociological terms, the concept of 'ideology' has been usurped. It no longer refers to a worldview dictated by vested interests, but to *any* worldview. Winlow et al. (2015: 18) develop this presciently:

> the grinding cynicism of the postmodern age exerts its influence on social experience, subjectivity and ideals. We must accept the continuation of the present as inevitable. The only cultural tools at hand to prevent us sinking into a bleak depression are irony, scepticism, cynicism and scorn. As compensation for our ongoing political complacency, we are granted leave to submerge ourselves in the shallow pleasantries of consumerised and mediatised culture. Our cynicism encourages us to believe all politicians are corrupt, greedy and self-interested. We assume that all of those at the fringes who are posing radical alternatives are in some way out for themselves.

Contemporary culture has been 'postmodernised' or 'relativised'; it is therefore, as Habermas (1989) argued, a neo-conservativist culture compatible with, if not simply willed or 'determined' by, the offspring of Mills's power elite.

Class-command dynamic

Pakulski and Waters (1996), among numerous others, announced the 'death of class' prematurely. The thesis on 'post-ideological relativity' effectively admits that *subjectively* class in financial capitalism is a less significant component of identity-formation than hitherto. *Objectively* it is a different story. Class relations, I maintain, now count for more, not less. Money, Habermas (1984, 1987) argues, is the steering medium of the economy, power that of the state. The American historian Landes (1998) succinctly averred that monied men (sic) have *always* bought men of power. Financial capitalism, to reiterate, bears testimony to a new class-command dynamic whereby ownership of capital buys power – in Britain and in the developed world – *on a scale beyond anything seen since the (twilight, land-owning, aristocratic) early decades of the twentieth century* (Piketty, 2014). This thesis is key for any revision of Mills's theory. Objectively, class relations have assumed a far greater significance even as, subjectively, their sway has diminished. To succeed materially, it has become more than advisable, and in fact a predictor of outcome, to inherit an advantage.

New inequality

The statistics of growing inequalities of wealth and income in Britain are almost as staggering as those in the USA. Under financial capitalism, wealth in general and income in particular have been taken from (a) the already impoverished 'have-nots' and (b) the 'squeezed middle', and donated to (c) the top 0.1% and (d) the other 99.9% of the top 10% and their allies from the non-squeezed or upper reaches of the middle class (Clark & Heath, 2014). Five British families, Oxfam (2014) has recently publicised, now have as much wealth as the poorest 20% of the population. As far as income is concerned, the CEOs of Britain's FTSEE 100 are now earning 143 times more than their staff. The likes of the wealth and income distributions marketed by the *Sunday Times* (Beresford, 2016), Piketty (2014) shows, seriously *under*-estimate the concentration of wealth. Table 3.2 summarises some representative data indicative of the quite extraordinary maldistribution of wealth and income in financial capitalism.

Prepotency of capital-ownership

The backlash against Piketty is in part explicable in terms of his exposure of the dearth of empirical support for neoliberalism's ideological thrust. His cautious and convincing case embarrasses those who privilege the privatization of public services and, as world-system therorist Wallerstein epitomised the capitalist 'project', the 'commodification of everything'. Piketty's prime equation picks up on and predicts the ascendancy of the return on capital versus wages in the present and for the foreseeable future: this is capitalism acting in accordance with rather than against its logic he argues. Inequality, as Adam Smith acknowledged in his *Wealth of Nations*, is capitalism's natural outcome and principal hazard. As far as financial capitalism is concerned, the boosted privileging of capital over wages underpins a new reinvigorated heritability of opportunity and outcome.

'High immorality'

Mills' notion of high immorality still resonates. I have argued elsewhere that those comprising the extreme or hard core of Clement and Miles' 'capitalist-executive' class, not the Occupy Movement's 1% *but the top 0.1%*, are – Habermas again – totally instrumental or strategic. As one financier was quoted as saying, 'what don't people understand? We don't do morality, we make money'. It is a feature of financial capitalism that 'making money' more readily trumps any communicative impetus to consensual, reciprocal community building. The system colonization of the lifeworld, *and those petit narratives that underpin and foster it* are gathering momentum.

Britain, I maintain, is currently ruled by a tiny class-driven political or command elite, 0.1% of its population or thereabouts, inviting a reference to a *governing oligarchy* (though Sayer (2015) prefers the term 'plutocracy'). As yet, this is a plausible but not corroborated contention. Before the argument is deepened, however, it will be helpful to reflect further on the concept of *elite*.

The term 'elite' typically refers to the incumbents of top positions in both the public and private sectors. The focus is on their individual characteristics. 'Vertical integration' refers to how representative they are of the total

Table 3.2 Inequalities of Wealth and Income in Financial Capitalism

---

Global Wealth

An Oxfam Report in 2016 found that the 62 richest billionaires in the world own
as much wealth as the poorer half of the world's population. One per cent of
the world's population owns more wealth than the other 99% combined.
The wealth of the poorest half of the world's population dropped by 41% between
2010 and 2015, despite an increase in the global population of 400m. In the same
period, the wealth of the richest 62 people increased by $500bn (£350bn) to $1.76tn.
Mark Goldring, the Oxfam GB chief executive said: 'world leaders' concern
about the escalating inequality crisis has so far not translated into concrete
action to ensure that those at the bottom get their fair share of economic
growth. In a world where one in nine people go to bed hungry every night, we
cannot afford to carry on giving the richest an ever bigger slice of the cake.

UK: Wealth and Income

In the UK, wealth is more evenly distributed than income. The richest 10% of
households hold 45% of all wealth. The poorest 50% own just 8.7%. This wealth
is unevenly spread across the UK. An average household in the South East has
almost twice the amount of wealth of an average household in Scotland.
The UK has a very high level of income inequality. Households in the bottom
10% of the population have on average a net income of £9,277. The top
10% have net incomes over nine times that (£83,897). Income inequality is
particularly stark at the top of the income scale, with the group with the ninth
highest incomes making only 60% of the top 10%'s income. Income inequality
is considerably higher with original than with net income, with the poorest
10% having an average original income of £4,467 whilst the top 10% have an
original income 24 times larger (£107,597).
Especially relevant to the analysis of the class/command dynamic in this volume,
the top 1% have incomes substantially higher than the rest of those in the top
10%. In 2012, the top 1% had an average income of £253,927 and the top 0.1%
had an average income of £919,882.
Moreover, a small all-male cadre of 'greedy bastards' at the top of the corporate
tree continues to be rewarded with ever-larger payments. In 2015, the bosses
of the UK's largest companies 'earned' an average of £5.5m (enjoying a 10%
pay rise). Advertising CEO Sir Martin Sorrell topped the high 'earners' league
for a second year, receiving a record £70m in 2015, one of the biggest annual
windfalls in UK corporate history.
The poorest 20% of households in the UK have only 8% of total income, whereas
the top 20% have 40%. As with wealth, there is considerable regional effect,
with London markedly in contrast with the North East.

UK: Changes Over Time

The UK became more equal in the postwar years of welfare statism. The share
of income going to the top 10% of the population fell over the 40 years to 1979
(from 34.6% in 1938 to 21% in 1979), while the share going to the bottom 10%
rose slightly. Income inequality grew significantly during the 1980s however,
peaking in 1990. Changes in income inequality have been less dramatic since.
Income inequality reached a new peak in 2009–2010, but fell back slightly and
has remained stable since. The financial crisis of 2008–2009 had little effect.
Income inequality in 2011–2012 was lower than before the recession: this was
due to falling incomes at the very top of the distribution and increases at the
very bottom, largely from social security payments.

By way of summary, in 2010, while the top 10% received 31% of all income, the bottom 10% received a mere 1%. In terms of wealth in the same year, 45% of all wealth in the UK was held by the richest 10%, the poorest 10% holding only 1%. Meanwhile, the top 1% did especially well, and the top 0.1% all but disappeared from view.

Source: The Equality Trust (2016a, 2016b).

population; 'horizontal integration' refers to their degree of connectivity and interaction (Dronkers & Schiff, 2007). Although this individualistic approach is paramount, more structural approaches are also to be found. Scott (2008: 32), for example, defines elites as 'those groups that hold or exercise domination within a society or within a particular area of social life'. He identifies four ideal types of elite. *Coercive* elites and *inducing* elites are rooted in allocative control over resources: they derive their power from the constraints that flow from the distribution of resources involved in 'force' and 'manipulation', respectively. The coercive elites are Pareto's 'lions', the inducing elites his 'foxes'. *Commanding* elites and *expert* elites owe their power to the discursive formation of legitimating and signifying principals and subalterns. Aping Pareto, Scott refers to these as 'bears' and 'owls', respectively.

To elaborate, coercive elites control access to the use of violence and can compel others into conformity, even to act against their wishes, desires and interests. Inducing elites exercise control via their financial and industrial capital, imposing conformity by influencing others' 'rational, self-interested calculations of personal or group advantage' (Scott, 2008: 33). Commanding elites comprise those who legitimately occupy top administrative positions in institutional hierarchies of management and control. Expert elites are those whose specialised, formal or arcane knowledge is contained in professional structures, affording them a generalised 'persuasive power'. Scott emphasises that these are ideal types and are rarely found in pure form.

So for Scott, elites denote membership of the most powerful positions in structures of domination. Elite members may or may not cohere into solidaristic groups. Elites, Scott argues, must be distinguished from classes (and statuses) *regardless of the degree of overlap in real situations.* He writes:

> 'economic elite' and 'capitalist class' … may be used interchangeably to describe various privileged, advantaged, or powerful economic groups. This tendency must be resisted if the analytical power of the elite concept is to be retained, as this is the only basis on which the dynamics of power can be clearly understood.
>
> (Scott, 2008: 34)

Scott's perspective on elites and classes is distinctively Weberian – via Weber's student Michels's interpretations of Pareto and Mosca.

Commenting on the recent Great British Class Survey, Savage (2015) has become increasingly attached to the notion of a 'wealth elite'. He discerns a growing polarization in financial capitalism between this elite and the 'precariat'. I accept the sociological utility of both terms. *But neither constitutes a 'class' in my book; and there's the rub.*

Although Scott (1991) has himself written on the 'ruling class', accounts of class-based rule are more often rooted in Marx than Weber. Marxist analysts now tend to be circumspect, sometimes studiously so. Erik Ohlin Wright is among the exceptions. I think it premature to abandon classical Marxian notions of class and class struggle. The distinction between capital ownership and wage labour still strikes me as pivotal, albeit in new and unanticipated structural and cultural contexts.

I lament the 'absence' from putative class schema of those whose ownership of capital buys more power from the state in post-1970s financial capitalism than could possibly have been foreseen during post-WW2 welfare capitalism. The less than 1% that comprised John Scott's 'ruling class' have always been able to hide in 'socio-economic classifications' like the RG, NS-SEC and the confused and confusing – because it conflates the material with the cultural – Great British Class Survey; hence the classification outlined in Table 3.1. Drawing on this table to pull a few threads together, in positing a revised class/command dynamic for financial capitalism I am claiming: (a) that a hard core of the capitalist executive, *most especially the 'capital monopolists'*, can now buy more power than hitherto from the state's power elite; and (b) that this is causally decisive for the maldistribution of health and longevity alluded to in Chapter 1. For me, Scott and Mills anticipate something of the class/command dynamic without nailing it: both, for all their perspicacity, and in their different ways, underestimate the continuity and tight(ening) Marxisant grip of objective class relations. New research shows that class has not lost its force, for all that the social environment in which it is compelling has shifted and diminished, demographically and as a result of top-down political party proformas like those of New Labour through the 1990s (Evans & Tilley, 2017).

Sociology and health inequalities

So how after all these preliminaries does financial capitalism's prepotent generative mechanism, the class/command dynamic, translate into a sociology of health inequalities? It does so via my *greedy bastards hypothesis* (or GBH). I had better explain, but without apologizing for its constituent terms. It takes a greedy bastard (GB) to privilege his (usually) or her (occasionally) nose in the trough of capital while many others plumb the social depths: a spade should be called a spade. The GBH asserts that the 'widening gap' and 'social gradient' exposed via the routine and regular deployment of socio-economic classifications like the RG and NS-SEC documented in Chapter 1, satisfy, even require, a retroductive inference to the impact of 'real' relations of class on the command relations of the state. Coburn (2009: 44) writes:

people with high SES (socio-economic status) do indeed live longer than those with less. SES, however, is a mere ranking of people according to income, educational attainment or occupational position. It reflects standards of living generally, and because these standards are related to many different types of disease, it is a good correlate of health status. But SES is itself a result of class forces. The nature of the capitalist class structure, and the outcome of class struggles, determine the extent and type of socio-economic inequalities in a given society, and the socio-economic inequalities in turn shape the pattern of health – and of health care. But while many theorists of the social determinants of health proclaim an interest in the basic determinants of health and health inequalities, much of their literature omits any consideration whatever of the political and class causes of SES and the SES-health relationship. When they speak of analyzing the 'causes' of disease, they seldom go far enough up the causal chain to confront the class forces and class struggles that are ultimately determinant.

(see also Scambler & Higgs, 2001)

Scambler & Scambler (2015: 342) develop this theme:

why buy power? The short answer through 'all' of capitalism's phases is to maximize the return on capital. The data from non- and post- as well as positivistic studies coalesce: increases in inequalities of wealth and income transmute into health inequalities, although the mechanisms remain obscure … inequalities are – above all else – the 'unintended consequences' of the wholly strategic behaviours of a hard core of the capital executive. The 'regressive' easing of the personal and corporate tax burdens on the 1 per cent, with which the four primary accountancy firms in Britain are complicit, is a form of symbolic violence. Via the decimation of trade union rights and the statutory safeguards and back-stops of wage-labour, free or cheap labour via internships, zero-hours contracts under-written by tax-payer benefits, outsourcing, benefit cuts inaccurately and misleadingly portrayed as austerity measures designed to cut what is actually a growing deficit, the closure and downgrading of final-salary pension schemes, and so on, the profits accruing to the few transmute into the disadvantage of many of the 99% +. The lining of the pockets of the less than 1 per cent kills people, especially within what contemporary positivists define as the bottom decile. Virschow and Engels were spot on.

I have cast a series of seven *asset flows* as the means by which the class relations that the GBH epitomises impact – via the command relations of the state – on health and longevity (i.e. constitute its 'media of enactment'). These are listed and briefly defined in Table 3.2. A few points of clarification are in order. First, as the Black Report decided a generation ago, the flow of material assets is prepotent for health and longevity. Second, as is implicit in the notion of 'flows', my argument is that people rarely either 'have' or 'do not have' assets known to be protective of or beneficial for health. Rather, these assets wax and wane, varying in strength over time. Third, there can be and often is compensation between asset flows. Thus, if someone is unexpectedly made redundant, the negative effect on that person's health via a diminished material asset flow might yet be mitigated by strong flows of biological, psychological or social assets. This is entirely consonant with socio-epidemiological and quantitative sociological research but is a conclusion often resisted by neo-positivists troubled by the daunting prospect of reducing 'flows' to variables. In fact, point four, both strong and weak flows tend to cluster: for example, a weak flow of material assets tends to be accompanied by weak flows of social, cultural, spatial and symbolic assets. Fifth, clustering is especially significant at critical points of the lifecourse, most especially in infancy and childhood, with ramifications for health well into adulthood. And sixth, people's 'subjective' readings of their asset flows can have an impact on their health independently of the 'objective' – in principle measurable – strength or weakness of flows (Marmot, 2004) (Table 3.3).

Consider the following 'fictional' illustrations of the pertinence and credibility of thinking in terms of asset flows. They are, I contend, in line with the considerable, cross-disciplinary and multifarious findings of research on health inequalities:

> Lilian is a 24-year old Afro-Caribbean who was brought up in Salford and who left school at 16. She moved to Lewisham in south London when she married aged 20. Her marriage broke down within a year and she is now reliant on state benefits to support her sons aged four and two in her privately rented one-bedroom flat. She feels insecure and fears a rent rise. Her flow of material assets, never strong, has weakened considerably. She remains isolated in Lewisham. She has no close friends: her social, cultural, symbolic and spatial assets are weak and/or weakened. But Lilian's hopes are still simmering: she is an aspiring writer who regularly turns out short stories, two of which have been published (one in the LRB). J.K. Rowling is her role model. Moreover, her family is known for its longevity, and all four grandparents – one pair in Manchester, the other in Trinidad – are in rude health. Her self-esteem has not been undermined. The flows of biological and psychological assets are strong, as is her (subjective) reading of her cultural and symbolic asset flows. So what price her health status and life expectancy? Might it be that a poor social prognosis will be annulled or even overturned by the happenstance of biological inheritance, talent and a fire that will not be dowsed?

> Steven's circumstances are quite different from Lilian's. He is a married senior lecturer in a well-known redbrick university aged 56 with a mortgage nearing completion, a good income and the prospect of a decent – if no longer final salary – pension scheme. His social, cultural, spatial and symbolic as well as his material asset flows are strong. But he has been

Table 3.3 Types of Asset Flow Salient for Health and Longevity

1 Biological (or body) assets can be affected by class relations even prior to birth. Low-income families, for example, are more likely to produce babies of low birthweight; and low birthweight babies carry an increased risk of chronic disease in childhood, possibly in part through biological programming;
2 Psychological assets yield a generalised capacity to cope, extending to what is increasingly conceptualised as 'resilience'. In many ways the 'vulnerability factors' that Brown and Harris (1978) found reduced working-class women's capacity to cope with life-events causally pertinent for clinical depression are class-induced interruptions to the flow of psychological assets;
3 Social assets have come to assume pride of place in many accounts of health inequalities and feature strongly in the work of Marmot and Wilkinson. The terms social assets or 'social capital' refer to aspects of social integration, networks and support. The political use to which social capital is being put should not occasion its neglect;
4 Cultural assets or 'cultural capital' are initially generated through processes of primary socialization and go on to encompass formal educational opportunities and attainment. Class-related early arrests to the flow of cultural assets can have long-term ramifications for employment, income levels, and therefore health;
5 Spatial assets have been shown to be significant for health by area-based studies. These have documented that areas of high mortality tend to be areas with high rates of net out-migration; and it tends to be the better qualified and more affluent who exercise the option to move;
6 Symbolic assets, representing the variable distribution of social status or 'honour', are known to impact on health via people's (sense of) social position, especially relative to those others who comprise their reference groups;
7 Material assets refer to 'relative deprivation' due to impoverishment and meagre standard of living. The relevance of material assets for health and longevity has long been stressed, although the mechanisms linking low income with health remain much debated.

Source: Scambler and Scambler (2015).

prescribed anti-depressants and has taken several periods of absence from work; he puts this down to stress. Seigrist would diagnose 'effort-reward imbalance': Steven feels his diligence and accomplishments are unrecognised by line-managers. Unlike Lilian, his self-esteem has taken a hit. His mother lived to 87, but his father's life was cut short by a heart attack at the age of 39. The question here is whether Steven's strong asset flows for health will be countermanded by a weak psychological and suspect biological asset flow. A keen cyclist, he might of course be run over by a heavy goods vehicle

Peter is 21 and has been living rough for 15 months. A regular truant from school, he ceased studying before 16. He left the parental home aged 20. His parents are both professionals, but he felt and was defined as a 'misfit' in his mid-teens; aged 19, a psychiatrist diagnosed borderline personality disorder. There is no history of psychiatric disorder in his family. He took soft drugs prior to experimenting with heroin and subsequently becoming a regular user at the age of 20. Peter's flows of health-enhancing assets have weakened dramatically over a short period. They are recoverable in principle but seem reliant on contingent events. Predictions are gloomy, not least because of an intense clustering of weak asset flows.

Shirley is 31 and finds it difficult to be optimistic about her future. She lives with her parents outside Newcastle. She is a heavy smoker. She has experienced several short-term relationships, but none have lasted beyond four months. She has a 'zero-hours' contract working in a supermarket. She has two close confidants from work. Her material asset flow derives from supportive parents and is as steady as it is challenging to her (subjective) sense of self-worth. Shirley's melancholic disposition deepened when her older sister died from breast cancer two years ago, at the age of 33, and her mother is currently undergoing treatment for the same condition. Her father works in the office of an estate agent. Shirley's biological, psychological, cultural and symbolic asset flows are weak, although the flows of spatial and, derivatively, material assets might offer limited compensation.

Summarizing at this point, there are specifiable components of a plausible sociology of health inequalities that might be condensed into eight propositions (see Scambler & Scambler, 2015: 4):

1   regimes of capital accumulation (involving relations of class) and their concomitant modes of regulation (involving relations of command) tend towards increasing inequalities of wealth and income even when flows of material assets are strengthening across populations as a whole;
2   the class/command dynamic in financial capitalism has seen a steep rise in material inequality, occasioned in significant part by the invigoration of class-based exploitation and state- or command-based oppression;
3   1 and 2 are pivotal for a viable sociology of health inequalities (and paradoxically explain why one is currently lacking in Britain and elsewhere);
4   the endlessly replicated statistical associations linking socio-economic classifications and alternate proxies for class with health and longevity, climaxing in the idea of the social gradient, bear testimony to the existence of real relations of class and to their causal efficacy;
5   neoliberalism's state-approved and policed policy of 'personal responsibility', sanctioned and foisted on the health domain via concepts like 'behavioural conditionality', affords ideological cover for 1 and 2;
6   Britain's health inequalities can be traced via financial capitalism's revised class/command dynamic back to the GBH;
7   though material assets remain crucial, other asset flows fuel the production and reproduction of health inequalities; and
8   it follows from 1 to 7 that the behaviours of the capital monopolists and power elite, representing financial capitalism's class/command dynamic, be defined as a critical 'social determinant of health', as *pathogenic*, and as worthy of study.

'Reforming' the National Health Service

Health care systems are clearly relevant for health status and longevity, although the link between 'good health care' and population health is more tenuous and complex than might be imagined. Britain was no pioneer of welfare or personal health care provision; on the contrary, it was a European laggard (see Scambler, 2002: 66–70; Scambler et al., 2014). The first direct engagement followed on from concerns about high rates of work absenteeism and lack of fitness for war duty among working men and resulted in the National Health Insurance Act of 1911. By means of Approved Societies, this legislation protected a segment of the *male* working class from the costs of sickness. The scheme drew in contributions from the state, employers and employees and entitled beneficiaries to free primary care by an approved panel doctor (that is, by a local general practitioner or GP) and to a sum of money to compensate for loss of earning power due to sickness. Better paid working men, women, children and older people were excluded and either had to opt for fee-for-service primary as well as secondary health care or fall back on a limited and fragmented system of 'public' (state-funded) or 'voluntary' (charitable) care. The Act covered 27% of the population in 1911, and this had only expanded to 45% by the beginning of WW2.

During the 1920s and 1930s, pressure grew to extend the reach of health care services. The resultant overhaul actually took place during WW2. It evolved out of Beveridge's (1942) painstaking blueprint for an all-out assault of the 'five giants' arresting social progress, namely, Want, Disease, Ignorance, Squalor and Idleness. The Beveridge Report incorporated plans for a National Health Service. The postwar displacement of Churchill's wartime government by Atlee's Labour Party, 1945–1951, witnessed not only the realization of the concept of the welfare state, but following the National Health Service (NHS) Act of 1946, a skillful piece of midwifery by Health Minister Aneurin Bevan, the birth of the NHS in 1948. Based on the principles of collectivism, comprehensiveness, universalism and equality (plus that of professional autonomy), the state was thenceforth committed to offer primary and secondary health care free at the point of service for anyone in need. Moreover, these services were to be funded almost exclusively out of central taxation.

The 1946 Act was a compromise with history and the medical profession. GPs escaped what they saw as salaried control and emerged as independent contractors paid capitation fees based on the number of patients on their books; the prestigious teaching hospitals won a substantial degree of autonomy; and GPs, and far more significantly hospital consultants, won the 'right' to continue to see patients privately. The survival of private practice was significant: 'the NHS was weakened by the fact that the nation's most wealthy and private citizens were not compelled to use it themselves and by the diluted commitment of those clinicians who provided treatment to them' (Doyal & Doyal, 1999: 364).

The consensus on the character of the NHS held steady through welfare capitalism, its initial 'tripartite' structure – involving divisions between GP, hospital and local authority services – surviving piecemeal social engineering. By the end of the 1960s, however, the growing number of people with long-term and disabling conditions in particular provoked calls for a more integrated as well as a more efficient and planned service. The result, in 1974, was a bureaucratic reorganization initiated by the Heath regime in 1974. Fourteen Regional Health Authorities (RHAs), 90 Area Health Authorities (AHAs) and 200 District Management Teams (DMTs) – concerned with planning, implementation and day-to-day management, respectively – were introduced and obliged to function by 'consensus management'. GPs remained independent contractors but were integrated at each level; and at each level there was a 'community health council' to act as a public watchdog. The Act also introduced a limited drug list for GPs to prescribe on the NHS and competitive tendering for support services (incorporating the private sector).

The 1970s recession that was to flick the switch to financial capitalism triggered a rethink about cost-containment in health care. In the first year of stability in spending, 1950–1951, the NHS had absorbed 4.1% of gross domestic product (GDP). This proportion fell steadily to 3.5% by the mid-1950s; by the mid-1960s it had regained and passed the level of 1950–1951; and by the mid-1970s it had risen to 5.7% of GDP. In fact, public expenditure as a whole reached a peak in 1975, accounting for nearly half of GDP.

The administrations headed by Wilson and Callaghan from 1974 to 1979 took steps to contain public expenditure, including that on health care. But when Thatcher was elected in 1979, she brought to office a set of convictions suited to the notion of a burgeoning crisis in welfare statism. She took full advantage of the fact that bureaucracies have long been easier to discern and condemn in the public than in the private sector (Galbraith, 1992). In 1983, Thatcher invited Roy Griffiths from Sainsbury's (where else?) to conduct an enquiry into NHS management structures. The result was an end to consensus management. A new hierarchy of managers on fixed-term contracts was imposed. From 1985 there was a general manager of the NHS itself and of each RHA and District Health Authority (DHA) (with DHAs replacing AHAs, which were abolished in 1982). These changes – towards a corporate style of management – also allowed for greater central control over all levels of activity, although the rationale for the 'new managerialism' was enhanced efficiency and cost-containment. NHS spending remained fairly constant through the 1980s at approximately 6.5% of GDP.

In 1988, amidst incessant politically motivated talk of crises of expenditure and delivery, Thatcher announced a comprehensive review of the NHS. The result was a White Paper, *Working for Patients*, published in 1989. This focused on the means of delivery of health care. It incorporated one of several of Thatcher's innovations to promote the private sector in the 1980s by introducing tax relief on private health insurance premiums for people aged over 60 years. The four principal proposals were: (a) the introduction of an 'internal' or quasi-market into the NHS; (b) additional provisions for professional accountability (most notably in relation to audit); (c) another streamlining of management along 'business lines'; and (d) the development of general practice (for instance, by altering GPs' contracts to foster activities like information-giving and screening, and by making it easier for patients to change GP).

The internal market was the most radical feature of the NHS and Community Care Act of 1990 that followed. It sat on a spectrum somewhere between a bureaucratic command and control economy and a private free market. If it was closer to the former, it was also a sign of things to come. The Act pioneered 'managed competition', which entailed a separation of the roles of 'purchaser' and 'provider'. DHAs became purchasers first and foremost, charged with buying primary and secondary services for their populations from providers in the public or private sectors. GP practices with more than 11,000 were 'encouraged' to become 'fundholders', permitted to buy diagnostic, outpatient and selected non-emergency surgical procedures for their patients from providers, including the private sector. Hospitals were similarly 'encouraged' to become self-governing NHS 'trusts' with greater managerial discretion. The income of these trusts would be based on their ability to market services to purchasers (i.e. to DHAs, fundholding GPs or private insurers). The political aspiration and agenda was obvious, yet the NHS was set to remain – if more in principle than practice – a centralised, tax-funded service accessible to all-comers on the basis of need and (largely) free at the point of use.

Thatcher's displacement by Major saw the introduction in 1992 of the Private Finance Initiative (PFI). This allowed for the private sector to build (and own) new hospitals and other health care facilities, which they then leased back to the NHS at often exorbitant rates on the back of 20–30 year deals. It was a convenient arrangement for the political elite since PFI building and refurbishment did not appear on government books (they represented an investment of private not public capital). By the time of Major's departure in 1997, expenditure on the NHS had topped 7% of GDP.

Blair and Brown lovingly embraced PFIs from 1997 to 2010. As Alyson Pollock (2005) presciently predicted, one day the chickens would come home to roost. And they have: PFIs are a major contributor to the indebtedness of many an NHS trust, the more so given the cuts or austerity measures following the financial crash. Disconcertingly, like his immediate Tory predecessors, Blair saw the welfare state as encouraging dependency, lowering self-esteem and undermining opportunity and responsibility. New Labour's 'third way' continued with and complemented Thatcher's experiment. An amended system of purchasing, or commissioning, was introduced via some 500 primary care groups (PCGs), evidence-based National Service Frameworks for major care areas and disease clusters were favoured, a National Institute for Clinical Excellence (NICE) to foster clinical guidelines and good practice in audit was established and a Commission for Health Improvement was set up to monitor the quality and delivery of services.

In 2000, faced with growing public concern, Blair undertook to raise spending on the NHS by 6.1% annually, in real terms, over a four-year period. In the same year he published 'The NHS Plan', which set service targets like reducing what Americans call 'queuing'. The Plan also announced: (a) a system of 'earned autonomy' designed to devolve power from central to local services; (b) 'modern contracts' for GPs and hospital doctors to reward quality and productivity (also to proscribe private work for newly qualified hospital consultants 'for perhaps seven years'; (c) the extension of prescribing rights to non-doctors; (d) a 'concordat' with private providers to optimise use of private facilities; and (e) new care trusts to commission health and social care under a single umbrella. These moves spoke of and promised continuity rather than discontinuity with Thatcher's project (indeed, Blair openly admired her).

The 2010 election resulted in a Cameron/Clegg coalition that backtracked on a (Tory) pre-election promise not to engage in a top-down reorganization of the NHS. Health Minister Andrew Lansley published a White Paper 'Liberating the NHS' only 60 days after the election. It was the product of protracted and insistent pre-election private sector lobbying. This was followed by the Health and Social Care Bill that opened the door for a root-and-branch privatisation of health care in England. It was a long, complex and devious Bill. There were five main 'rhetorical' themes: strengthening commissioning services, increasing democratic accountability and public voice, liberating provision of health services, strengthening public health services and reforming health and social care's arm's length bodies. This was the coating of sugar to disguise an otherwise distasteful product.

Five specific organizational changes were mooted: by April of 2013, the extant 192 primary care trusts would be abolished and GPs would join commissioning consortia, these consortia would control 80% of the NHS budget, services would be purchased from 'any willing provider', all NHS hospitals would become foundation trusts by 2014 and commissioning would be overseen by an NHS 'financial regulator', *Monitor*. Some critics were not fooled. Why would the new commissioning consortia function better than primary care trust commissioning? What would the role of private companies be with regard to commissioning criteria? What would be the role of *Monitor* in European law? How would patients have 'more choice'? Where would the efficiency savings come from? Would the pursuit of efficiency savings be at the expense of quality?

A period of 'consultation' and debate was extended. The medical profession, a reluctant recruit to the original concept of an NHS, questioned and subsequently opposed the Bill. Then it folded. Doctors' professional bodies, it seemed, were ready to take industrial action to defend pay and conditions but not to safeguard a public NHS. Public protests were similarly ineffective, and the Bill became an Act in March of 2012. Later in 2012, the coalition pushed a (strategically re-written but equivalent) 'regulation 75' through the Houses of Parliament, removing residual obstacles to the unfettered promotion of for-profit health care.

A number of preliminary comments are in order. Neither the Tories nor the Liberal Democrats who joined them in an unlikely coalition had a mandate to 'reform' the NHS in the way they did. Moreover, it was a reform carried out against the background of Brown's efficiency savings announced in mid-2009 and amounting to £15–20bn in three years starting April 2011. The reform was opposed by the medical, nursing and other health professions, polls showed widespread public concern and a series of campaigns and protests were sidelined and ignored. Although a small number of health professionals and academics were recruited to the coalition cause, there is no doubt that 'best evidence' on comparative health care bore testimony to the regressive nature of the Health and Social Care Bill/Act: this was policy-based evidence, not evidence-based policy. Finally, it emerged later that for-profit providers were not only lobbying the Tories before the election but were intimately involved in the thrust and composition of the Bill (e.g. via the Future Forum). They were lining up to takeover NHS services. The leading private providers – H5, accounting for 80% of private hospitals and 85% of private beds – had formed an alliance as early as December 2010. Much of this clandestine activity was wrongly portrayed as 'internal to the NHS' rather than as external lobbying (see Leys & Player, 2011).

At the time of writing, we are already experiencing the predictable short-term effects of the Health and Social Care Act, with ill-equipped and predatory for-profit providers taking over services and cashing in on the NHS 'brand'. The 'revolving door' is also well oiled. Alex Scott-Samuel (2012) has taken a medium to long-term view, anticipating that: the NHS will become a subcontracting operation privileging competing private providers; that services of 'low clinical priority' will cease to be free; that a market for health insurance will emerge, affordable only for the affluent, which will drive up costs (administrative, fees, private profits); and that the development of personal health budgets will lead to personal charges as commissioning groups come to operate on an individual basis in order to be compatible with the insurance companies (i.e. an end to 'population-based pooling of risk'). The Health and Social Care Act was always going to be, and is, a profoundly regressive piece of legislation for which the British Medical Association (BMA) in particular was a shameful accomplice. PFI debt, cuts and privatisation are destroying perhaps the most just, efficient and effective – if of course imperfect – health care system in the developed world.

What do the data tell us at the time of writing, even as May takes over from Cameron? A number of things are already clear in this early transitional period of cutting-to-privatisation:

- privatised health care augments costs, requiring an expanded bureaucracy that comes with contracts, billing and litigation (the USA has the highest proportion of private provision and its total (non-universal) health care costs now exceed 16% of GDP, compared with Britain's nearly 9% (it was 5%–6% when Thatcher was elected);

- privatisation encourages cherry-picking, whereby the private sector takes on the more lucrative work (e.g. hip and knee replacements), leaving the NHS to deal with the rest;
- fees creep in as NHS services are cut and hospitals are pushed into greater debt, leading to mergers, closures or for-profit providers coming to the rescue (like Circle has at Hinchingbrooke);
- quality of care is sacrificed to cost (e.g. Serco's failure to deliver an out-of-hours GP service in Cornwall);
- rationing grows, affording a trigger for patients to 'go private' (more than a half of NHS trusts are already rationing treatments);
- 'commercial accountability' makes it impossible to properly scrutinise public spending via contracts with for-profit providers focused primarily on their shareholders;
- privatisation leads to a fragmentation of the health service as services are re-fashioned according to market principles.

At the time of writing, some three years after the passing of the Health and Social Care Act, Virgin Care runs 358 GP surgeries, provides 100 plus services across the country and is currently (in 2017) going to court about not being awarded an NHS contract. Serco has won a £140m contract to run community health care in Suffolk and, most unhappily, the £32m contract to run out-of-hours GP services in Cornwall mentioned above. Sainsbury's now has over 260 pharmacies across the UK. Specsavers, the optometrists and eye wear specialists based in the tax haven of Guernsey, has been awarded more than 30 contracts to supply hearing aids and community audiology services on high streets across the country. I could go on. In the meantime, people are waiting longer in hospital accident and emergency departments and operations are being cancelled daily even as Tory Secretary of State Jeremy Hunt, long committed to the privatisation of the NHS, attempts to impose junior doctor contracts as part and parcel of a plan to deliver a 24/7 service beyond the one he inherited. Tory MPs filibustered an attempt to introduce a private member's National Health Service Bill to reverse the privatisation of the NHS in March of 2016.

So why has all this taken place? It seems clear enough. The capital monopolists and their principal allies, the auxiliaries and sleepers, who fuel our governing oligarchy or plutocracy – that is, those who buy, hold and use power to their pecuniary advantage – have sufficient sway in financial capitalism to open up *even* the NHS for profiteering. Thatcher prepared the ground, but Cameron and May have been able to go further. The privatisation of the NHS and the likely commodification of health care might have been halted by a BMA-led campaign provoking a crisis of legtimation for the power elite, but that opportunity was lost. We need to recognise that if capital can purchase enough power, it will pursue accumulation. It is once again a class/command issue. If this sociological/structural dimension is ignored, we become ideological co-optees and deny ourselves the theoretical capacity to explain and counter regressive policies. To paraphrase Bill Clinton, 'it's class warfare, stupid'.

In sum, even as the class/command dynamic is causally critical for the social determinants of health and life expectancy, so it is for the nature of the health care system. Moreover, if its salience for the former is incidental – the GBs comprising the hard core of the capital executive do not set out to kill people by strangling their asset flows (homicide), even if the blinkered pursuit of their vested interests and the covering ideology of neoliberalism have that effect (manslaughter) – its salience for the latter is unambiguous. The NHS in England is being coldly and calculatingly broken up and sold off to line pockets: there is a better case for homicide here, for example, when a privatised ambulance service is demonstrably slow to respond to emergency calls and delivers charges too late to under-staffed and overly distant hospital accident and emergency departments as a direct and predictable result of a mix of PFI-occasioned and other funding cuts, closures and privatisations *and is re-awarded the contract.*

4 Archer, reflexivity and middle-range theories

The focus hitherto has been on the ways in which real social structures and relations, particularly those of class and state, can and do creep up on individuals to fabricate, nudge and occasionally coerce them into milieux, circumstances and even behaviours beyond their ken *and that can and do circumscribe and even shorten their lives*. In this chapter, attention switches to the causal efficacy and real, if limited, potency of agency. Bhaskar championed the causal power of agency, but Archer has developed Bhaskar's transformational model in an explicitly sociological direction via her exploration of reflexivity. Archer's notion of the 'morphogenetic society' is discussed in Chapter 6, so an extended reference to her evolving oeuvre here is warranted (I draw here on Block et al., 2017).

Archer has always been concerned with the relations between *structure* and *agency*. It is an interest that can be traced back to her time as a post-doctoral student at the Sorbonne, which coincided with the explosive events of 1968. Part of Bourdieu's team, her early research focused on a comparative study of national education systems. Her *Social Origins of Educational Systems*, published in 1979, broke new ground and has been a catalyst for subsequent macro-analyses. Her core claim was that centralization was crucial in accounting for what happened in French education, and decentralization no less crucial in accounting for what happened in British education. How did the former come to be centralised, she asked, and the latter decentralised?

She argued that prior to the emergence of state systems of education, the church played a pivotal and dominant role both in terms of resources and in terms of curricula. Education was in this sense 'mono-integrated' with the church. In the event of increasing state intervention, however, this mono-integration was displaced by 'multi-integration' with a plurality of institutions. State intervention and its concomitant multi-integration have characterised the (less constrained) British education system far more than its (more constrained) French counterpart.

Archer presented each of centralization and decentralization as 'emergent properties', highlighting the ways the different parts of each system are linked together. She also introduced her 'morphogenetic approach'. The transition prompted by state intervention in education comprised a 'morphogenetic cycle'. Structural conditioning (which is temporally prior, relatively autonomous yet possessive of causal powers), she maintained, conditions social interaction, which in its turn generates structural elaboration. This scheme – structural conditioning underlying/leading to social interaction underlying/leading to structural elaboration – has underpinned all her subsequent writings.

Archer (2007a: 38) later reflected further on where state education systems came from and what novel causal powers they exerted after their elaboration, writing:

> these powers work as underlying generative mechanisms, producing empirical tendencies in relation to 'who' gained access to education, 'what' constituted the definition of instruction, 'which' processes became responsible for subsequent educational change, and 'how' those ensuing changes were patterned. Crucially, the answers to all these questions differed according to the 'centralised' or 'decentralised' structuring of the new educational systems. This raised a major philosophical problem. It was being claimed that educational systems possessed properties emergent from the relations between their parts – summarized as centralization and decentralisation – that exercised causal powers. However, these two properties could not be attributes of people, who cannot be centralized or decentralized, just as no system can possess the reflexivity, intentionality and commitment of the agents whose actions first produced and then continuously sustained these forms of state education.

Her agenda was set.

Archer (1988) went on to conceptualise 'culture' as an objective phenomenon (akin to Popper's 'World Three'). In this way, she distinguished between the ontological status of culture and what people and/or groups make of it epistemologically. Culture, for her, is therefore not a 'community of shared meanings'; rather, there exists a 'cultural system' ('replete with complementarities and contradictions'). There is also 'socio-cultural interaction', according to which groups draw and elaborate upon components of the cultural system in line with their interests and projects.

Archer (1995) sought to establish a credible and 'useable' framework for conducting substantive sociological research. In the process, she noted that social theory – including critical realism – had committed far more energy to articulating how structural and cultural properties are transmitted to agents and shape their thoughts, beliefs, values and actions than to how these properties are accommodated and dealt with, sometimes innovatively, by agents.

She noted that causal efficacy has tended (a) to be granted *either* to structure *or* to agency and (b) to be granted more often to structure than to agency. She deployed and critiqued the notion of 'conflation'. She maintained that the denial of autonomy to agency (or 'downwards conflation') has far exceeded the denial of autonomy to structure (or 'upwards conflation'). An alternative account to be found in the sociological literature, for example in the work of Giddens, holds that structure and agency are 'co-constitutive', that is, structure is reproduced through agency but is simultaneously constrained and enabled by structure ('central conflation'). Archer rejects not only downwards and upwards but also central conflation. Conflationary approaches, she contends, preclude sociological investigation of the relative influence of each of structure and agency.

The approach associated with both her early and later labours on the relationship between structure and agency is epitomised in the term 'analytic dualism'. Like Bhaskar, she reinforces the interdependence between structure and agency. At any given time, antecedently existing structures constrain and enable agents, whose actions produce intended and unintended consequences, which reproduce (*morphostasis*) or transform (*morphogenesis*) these structures. What she adds is a timeline, as in the formula rehearsed above: structural conditioning underlying/*leading to* social interaction underlying/*leading to* structural elaboration. She refers to *morphogenetic sequences*. It is important to spell out what this amounts to, given its centrality to Archer theory. To reiterate, at any given moment in time, antecedently existing structures constrain and enable agents, whose actions deliver intended and unintended consequences, which lead in turn to structural elaboration and the reproduction or transformation of the existing structures. In the same vein, the initially antecedent structures were themselves the product of structural elaboration resulting from the actions of prior agents. Archer argues that this scheme – of morphogenetic sequences – permits, via the isolation of those structural and/or cultural factors that afford a context of action for agents, the investigation of how those factors mould the subsequent interactions of agents and how those interactions in turn reproduce or transform the initial context. Social processes are of course comprised of many such sequences. However, their temporal ordering allows for an examination of the internal causal dynamics of each sequence. In this way, it is possible to give *empirical* (as opposed to purely theoretical) accounts of how structural and agential phenomena interlink over time. The central thesis in the present contribution might be understood in terms of morphogenetic sequences that give rise to health inequalities.

Archer (2000) has contested sociological imperialism in all of its many guises (most recently, social constructionism, see Chapter 2). The 'person', she insisted, cannot be portrayed 'as society's gift'. *Being Human* did not turn its back on structure and culture; rather, it offered a reconceptualisation of human beings:

> each and every one of us has to develop a (working) relationship with every order of natural reality: nature, practice and the social. Distinctions between the natural, practical and social orders are real, although it is usually the case that they can only be grasped analytically because they are subject to considerable empirical superimposition. Nevertheless,

that does not preclude the fact that human subjects confront dilemmas, which are different in kind, when encountering each of the three orders. Neither does it diminish the fact that it is imperative for human survival to establish sustainable and sustaining relations with each.

(Archer, 2007a: 39)

Sociology, to reiterate once more, cannot wrap everything up.

Archer pinpoints *Being Human* as 'pivotal'. In it, she conceptualises unique human persons. No society or social organization possesses self-awareness; but each and every human being does. What difference, then, does this self-awareness make to the nature of the social? Archer's analytic dualism comes into play here. Only if the distinction between structure and agency (and indeed between objectivity and subjectivity) is upheld can it be acknowledged that humans can and do reflexively examine their personal concerns in the light of their social circumstances and can and do evaluate their social circumstances in the light of their concerns (Archer, 2007a: 41).

Structure, Agency and the Internal Conversation, published in 2003, moved this analysis of human reflexivity on. In it, Archer maintains that personal reflexivity mediates the effects of objective social forms on us. It helps us understand *how* structure influences agency. With customary clarity, Archer writes:

> reflexivity performs this mediatory role by virtue of the fact that we deliberate about ourselves in relation to the social situations that we confront, certainly fallibly, certainly incompletely and necessarily under our own descriptions, because that is the only way we can know anything. To consider human reflexivity play that role of mediation also means entertaining the fact that we are dealing with two ontologies: the objective pertaining to social emergent properties and the subjective pertaining to agential emergent properties. What is entailed by the above is that subjectivity is not only (a) real, but (b) irreducible, and (c) that it possesses causal efficacy.

(2007a: 42; see also Archer, 2007b)

It is the 'internal conversation' that denotes the manner in which humans reflexively make their way in the world. This inner dialogue about self-in-society, and *vice versa*, is what makes most of us 'active', as opposed to 'passive', agents. Being an active agent involves defining, refining and prioritizing concerns and elaborating projects out of them. In so far as these projects are successful, constellations of concerns translate into a set of practices. This set of practices constitutes a personal modus vivendi. So, *concerns lead to projects lead to practices.* Decrying any form of idealism, Archer adds that concerns can be ignoble, projects illegal and practices illegitimate! What people are doing in the course of their internal conversations is shaping themselves and contributing to the reshaping of the social world.

Reflexivity does not reduce to one homogeneous mode of deliberation. Rather, it is exercised through different modalities. Archer discerns three 'dominant modalities': *Communicative, Autonomous* and *Meta-Reflexivity*. The dominance of any one of these derives from their relationship to their natal context in conjunction with their personal concerns.

Archer (2007c) offers the following definitions of her three principal modes of reflexivity:

- The communicative reflexives are those whose internal conversations require completion and confirmation by others before resulting in a course action;
- The autonomous reflexives are those who sustain self-contained internal conversations, leading directly to action;
- The meta-reflexives are those who are critically reflexive about their own internal conversations and critical too about effective action in society.

Considered as generative mechanisms, these different dominant modes of reflexivity have what Archer calls 'internal consequences' for their practitioners as well as 'external consequences for society'. Internally, Archer found from a small-scale study oriented to social mobility that communicative reflexivity is associated with social immobility, autonomous reflexivity with upward social mobility and meta-reflexivity with social volatility. Externally, communicative reflexives contribute to social stability and integration through their 'evasion' of constraints and enablements, their endorsing of their natal contexts and their active forging of a dense micro-world that reconstitutes their 'contextual continuity' and projects it into the future. By contrast, the autonomous reflexives act strategically, in Archer's words, by 'avoiding society's snakes to ride up its ladders' (Archer, 2007a: 43). They represent 'contextual discontinuity'. The meta-reflexives are society's 'subversive agents', immune alike from the rewards and blandishments linked to enablements and the forfeits associated with constraints. They act out Weber's 'value rationality' amidst the 'contextual incongruity' that shaped their lives. They are a source of counter-cultural values, inclined to context both oppressive moves on the part of the state and exploitation arising from the economy.

The themes addressed here are picked up in Archer's (2012) *Reflexive Imperative*. She argues that society is currently being rapidly reshaped and distanced from modernity; she highlights in particular a new global realm of 'opportunities', as well as enhanced migration, increased education and a proliferation of novel skills, not to mention the changing nature of reflexivity itself. All this suggests a move away from communicative reflexivity, which is associated with traditionalism, towards autonomous reflexivity, which is apt and ripe for global opportunities, with meta-reflexivity producing 'patrons of a new civil society expressive of humanistic values'.

This move towards what Archer calls *morphogenetic society* jettisons some citizens. The logic and global reach of opportunity require the continuous revision of personal projects and serve as obstacles to any settled modus vivendi. The reflexivity of some, maybe many, becomes 'fractured' as a consequence.

- The fractured reflexives are those whose internal conversations intensify their distress and disorientation rather than leading to purposeful courses of action.

It is the communicative reflexives who are most fragile and vulnerable to displacement into the category of fractured reflexive (the majority of fractured reflexives in Archer's own investigation started out as communicative reflexives).

Archer's current work is focused around the notion of morphogenetic society. Partial morphostasis has yielded to untrammelled morphogenesis. This does not mean that she signs up – with Beck, Bauman and others – to the displacement or circumvention of social structure: there is never a non-structured social world. But she does detect a considerable social shift. Such shifts – for agents and social structures alike – occur in interlocking and temporally complex ways. Agents are formed in contexts set by social structural parameters (embracing language-games, norms, communities, power relations and so on). On an altogether different timescale, the structures themselves change as a result of the choices and activities of historically situated agents. The result is a series of cycles with different timelines. Back to a familiar 'formula': structural conditioning > social interaction > structural elaboration.

So what morphogenatic sequences or cycles and generative mechanisms are presently at work? Social morphogenesis, Archer confesses, is an umbrella concept, '*whereas any generative mechanism is a particular that needs identifying, describing and explaining* – by its own analytical history of emergence' (Archer, 2014: 95). She specifies three orders of emergent properties. Thus:

> the three coincide with what are conventionally known as the micro-, meso- and macro-levels: dealing respectively with the situated action of persons or small groups, because there is no such thing as contextless action; with 'social institutions', the conventional label for organizations with a particular remit, such as government, health, education etc at the meso-level; and with the relation between structure and culture at the most macroscopic level.
>
> (Archer, 2014: 95)

Archer's argument starts at the macro-level, but with the important rider that each – macro-, meso- and micro-level – stratum is 'activity-dependent' on that or those beneath it and that both 'downwards' and 'upwards' causation are continuous and intertwined.

Society for Archer comprises the relations between 'structure' and 'culture'. Society is the consequence of *relations between relations*, all of which are ever activity-dependent. Structures are primarily materially based, cultures primarily ideational. In a nutshell, Archer contends that in what she terms 'late modernity', the interplay between economic competition and technological diffusion has fuelled intensified morphogenesis across the whole array of social institutions. At the same time, it has rapidly augmented the cultural system. Thus, the two – structural and cultural – constituents of the generative mechanism have: (a) themselves undergone morphogenesis, and (b) their synergy has extended this to the rest of the social order via knock-on effects (Archer, 2014).

Archer does not proclaim the arrival of morphogenetic society, nor does she furnish a 'manifesto for morphogenetic society' (Archer, 2013). Although both structure and culture in late modernity can be said to promote morphogenesis, they nevertheless issue in different and contrasting 'situational logics of action'. The for-profit market sector would extend the *logic of competition* throughout the social order, embracing schools, universities, hospitals and so on. But scientific and technological 'diffusionsists' are committed to a *logic of opportunity* and so are hostile to bureaucratic regulation and restricted access; outcomes are not assessed according to the criterion of profitability. This tension between structure and culture – discordance between logics – has given rise to a 'relationally contested order'. The generative mechanism of 'competition-diffusion' is extremely morphogenetic, but no social transformation is imminent. We may, Archer avers, have to live with gradualism for a while. Ending on a marginally more optimistic note, Archer (2014: 115) suggests that diffusionist agencies might yet become the research and development department for a future civil society and civil economy.

> Their interim task is to make the 'logic of opportunity' more wide-reaching within economic activity and to demonstrate that incremental increases in socially useful value and augmentation of the commons are contributions to the common good that are genuinely beneficial to all – thus illustrating that win-win outcomes are realistic goals for the social order. That alone grounds optimism about gradualism leading to the transformation of global society.

Reframed in Archer's analysis and timeline for change are Dawe's 'two sociologies': on opposite ends of the spectrum, structural-functionalsists like Parsons *and* interactionists, phenomenologists and ethnomethodologists like Blumer, Schutz and Garfinkel (see Chapter 2). Archer argues that her scheme of morphogenetic sequences permits, via the isolation of those structural and/or cultural factors that afford a context for action for agents, the investigation of how those factors shape the subsequent interactions of agents and how those interactions in turn reproduce or transform the initial context. Social processes are comprised of many such sequences. Yet, their temporal ordering allows for a probing of the internal causal dynamics of each sequence. In this way, it is possible to give empirical – rather than purely theoretical – accounts of how structural and agential phenomena interlink over time.

In her *Being Human* (2000), Archer argued, against the likes of social constructionists, that the 'person' is not 'society's gift'. She proffered a reconceptualisation of what it is to be human:

> each and every one of us has to develop a (working) relationship with every order of natural reality: nature, practice and the social. Distinctions between the natural, practical and social orders are real, although it is usually the case that they can only be grasped analytically because they are subject to considerable empirical superimposition. Nevertheless, that does not preclude the fact that human subjects confront dilemmas, which are different in kind, when encountering each of the three orders. Neither does it diminish the fact that it is imperative for human survival to establish sustainable and sustaining relations with each.
>
> (Archer, 2000: 39)

Sociology can no more finalise or *wrap up* explanations of health inequalities than it can explanations of who has recurrent epileptic seizures and why.

No society, Archer argues, possesses self-awareness; but each human does. What difference does this self-awareness make to the nature of the social? Here, Archer's analytic dualism comes into play. Only if the distinction between structure and agency – as well, in fact, as that between objectivity and subjectivity – is maintained can it be recognised that humans can and do evaluate their social circumstances and that they can and do evaluate their circumstances in the light of their concerns (Archer, 2007a: 41).

Reflexivity mediates the effects of objective social forms. It facilitates our understanding of 'how' structure influences agency. Thus:

> reflexivity performs this mediatory role by virtue of the fact that we deliberate about ourselves in relation to the social situations that we confront, certainly fallibly, certainly incompletely and necessarily under our own descriptions, because that is the only way we can know anything. To consider human reflexivity plays that role of mediation also means entertaining the fact that we are dealing with two ontologies: the objective pertaining to social emergent properties and the subjective pertaining to agential emergent properties. What is entailed by the above is that subjectivity is not only (a) real, but (b) irreducible, and (c) that it possesses causal efficacy.
>
> (Archer, 2007a: 42; see also Archer, 2007b and Brock et al., 2017)

Agency is necessarily contextualised, and Archer offers a three-stage model to address this (see Table 4.1). Vygotsky (1934) argued that while external speech is for others, 'inner speech' is for oneself. Archer defends this notion of an 'internal conversation'. She maintains that:

Table 4.1 Archer's Three-Stage Model

1 Structural and cultural properties *objectively* shape the situations that agents confront involuntarily, and inter alia possess generative powers of constraint and enablement in relation to
2 the subject's own constellations of concerns, as *subjectively* defined in relation to the three orders of natural reality: nature, practice and the social.
3 Courses of action are produced through the *reflexive deliberations* of subjects who *subjectively* determine their practical projects in relation to their objective circumstances.

Source: Archer (2007a); and see Scambler (2012b).

- it is a genuinely *interior* phenomenon, and one that underwrites the private life of the social subject;
- its subjectivity has a first-person ontology, precluding any attempt to render it in the third-person; and
- it possesses causal efficacy.

She (2007c: 66) builds on this model via a 'guiding hypothesis', namely, that 'the interplay between people's nascent 'concerns' (the importance of what they care about) and their 'context' (the continuity or discontinuity of their social environment) shapes the mode of reflexivity they regularly practice.'

To reiterate, Archer discerns four principal ideal types of reflexivity. These are summarised in Table 4.2 (see also Scambler, 2012b). We all engage, she suggests, in communicative reflexivity, but only for some does it become the dominant mode of reflexivity. What is distinctive about the internal conversation of *communicative reflexives* is that its conclusion requires the input of others: intra-subjectivity needs to be supplemented by inter-subjectivity (Archer, 2007c: 102). Given our natal or initially 'involuntary' placement in society, these 'others' are typically recruited from those comprising communicative reflexives' local peers or reference groups (hence in Archer's pilot investigations, there is a tendency to social immobility).

By contrast, the internal conversations of *autonomous reflexives* are self-contained affairs. The lone inner dialogue is sufficient to determine a course of action. When this is the dominant mode of reflexivity, those involved neither seek nor need the involvement of others to inform their decision-making. Naturally, autonomous reflexives also engage in communicative reflexivity, but this for them is not strictly necessary. 'Whilst the autonomous subject may respond readily, articulately and take an interest in the reactions of others, none of these interchanges is driven by need' (Archer, 2007c: 114).

Meta-reflexives' internal conversations involve routines of self-questioning. 'Why did I say that?' 'Why am I so reticent to say what I think?' Meta-reflexives are conversant with their own reflexivity and are typically preoccupied with the moral standing or worth of their projects and their worthiness to undertake them.

Table 4.2 Archer's Modes of Reflexivity

Modes	Description
Communicative reflexives	Those whose internal conversations require completion and confirmation by others before resulting in courses of action.
Autonomous reflexives	Those who sustain self-contained internal conversations, leading directly to action.
Meta-reflexives	Those who are critically reflexive about their own internal conversations and critical about effective action in society.
Fractured reflexives	Those whose internal conversations intensify their distress and disorientation rather than leading to purposeful courses of action.

Source: Archer (2007c).

Fractured reflexives are accorded a separate and extended treatment. Fractured reflexivity lends itself to passive agency, unlike the other trio of ideal types. For them, internal conversations typically lead to disorientation and distress: their deliberations go round in circles and lack conclusions. Communicative reflexives are particularly vulnerable to displacement into the category of fractured reflexive (the majority of fractured reflexives in Archer's sample started out as communicative reflexives).

Deploying the terminology of Habermas (1984, 1987), it might be said that communicative reflexives are (communicatively) oriented to consensus, autonomous reflexives are (strategically) oriented to outcome, meta-reflexives are oriented to values and fractured reflexives are non- or disoriented.

Agency, reflexivity and health inequalities

Focused autonomous reflexives

The principal message in Archer's discussion is that, considered as generative mechanisms, the four different modes of reflexivity have 'internal consequences' for their practitioners as well as 'external consequences for society'. I have argued that the GBs comprising the governing oligarchy or plutocracy in financial capitalism, core actors in its class/command dynamic, display many of the characteristics of autonomous reflexivity. I have accorded them their own sub-category, referring to them as *focused autonomous reflexives* (Scambler, 2012b). Before I expand on this, a few preliminary comments are in order.

The first draws on a distinction between stigma, denoting an infringement against norms of shame, and deviance, denoting an infringement against norms of blame (Scambler, 2009). The sole reason 'benefit cheats' are effectively so portrayed by the governing oligarchy and mainstream media – that is, shamed *and blamed* (for their shame) by *the tax-avoiding/tax evading GBs featuring in my GBH* – is that the latter possess the capital and power to make their charges plausible and 'stickable' while the former do not (Link & Phelan, 2001). As most conspicuously shown by the bankers in the aftermath of 2008–2009, the GBs can get away with almost anything without being effectively shamed or blamed. By what criteria, for example, was it ever acceptable for the late Duke Of Westminster, or indeed now his son, to inherit the means to forego labour entirely while others born less privileged *must*, on pain of financial retribution, respond positively to an 'imperative to work' sponsored and policed by the governing oligarchy? 'Excusing conditions' are rarely sought from the oligarchy in a post-Fordist, post-welfare statist and postmodern or relativised culture that allows neoliberal ideology to function as a default petit narrative (Scambler, 2002, 2012b). To reiterate Habermas's (1989) observation, a postmodern, relativised culture is intrinsically conservative. Nor, harking back to Wright Mills, does the governing oligarchy as a whole need to 'conspire' often: Mills's 'tacit understanding' suffices.

The second point is a crucial one. It has been suggested that (a) my reference to the greedy bastards who comprise the class-based constituents of the governing oligarchy, and (b) my deployment of Archer's writings on reflexivity and internal conversations, serve to *individualise* what are essentially social relations. This is to misread my thesis. I have always insisted both that those I shall characterise as focused autonomous reflexives are eminently replaceable – rather than uniquely gifted or charismatic – and that they are mere 'surfers' of social structures and relations of class and command. *They are delivered by a compound of generative mechanisms and of tendencies.*

Third, and once again treading in the footsteps of Habermas (1984, 1987), I am positing a learned predisposition to strategic as opposed to communicative action on the part of the GBs:

> Habermas argues that in modern, highly differentiated societies 'system' (economy and state) and 'lifeworld' (private/household and public/deliberative spheres) have become 'de-coupled'; and the former, via their 'steering media' of money and power, have increasingly come to dominate or 'colonize' the latter … In the less complex era of 'The Prince', Machiavelli discerned an incompatibility between the goals and practices of the statesman and the (Christian) moralist. In contemporary Habermasian terms, the former was essentially strategic, the latter essentially communicative.
>
> (Scambler, 2012b: 143)

My focused autonomous reflexives are likewise 'essentially strategic'. Their bias to outcomes via their fixations on money (capital) and power neuter any residual commitments to consensus: morality survives only as a strategic issue, subordinate to short-term financial, business or political agendas.

Table 4.3 outlines my ideal type of the focused autonomous reflexive. To leave no ambiguity, neither the GBs nor those comprising the power elite, who

Table 4.3 Attributes of the Focused Autonomous Reflexive

Total commitment
The focused autonomous reflexive (FAR) exhibits an overriding engagement with
  accumulating capital (and personal wealth/income) or and/or power. Nothing
  less will suffice: that is, any deficit in commitment will result in absolute or
  relative failure.

Nietzschean instinct
Born of a Hobbesian notion of the natural human state, or of human nature, the
  commitment of the FAR betrays a ruthless determination to cut every corner
  necessary to win an advantage over rivals.

Fundamentalist ideology
The commitment of the FAR is not only total and Nietzschean but
  fundamentalist: it does not admit of compromise. It is an ideology – that is, a
  standpoint emerging from a coherent set of vested (class/command) interests –
  that cannot brook or tolerate alternatives.

Cognitive insurance
While cognitive dissonance is (near) universal, the governing oligarchy is able,
  courtesy of the new class/command dynamic, to take out enough insurance
  to draw its sting. Accusations of greed, excess and irresponsibility are rarely
  internalised. Such epistemological and ontological security is the exception
  rather than the rule in financial capitalism.

Tunnel vision
A concomitant of a total, Nietzschean and fundamentalist commitment is the
  sidelining of other matters and a reflex and frequently gendered delegation of
  these to others to sort.

Lifeworld detachment
The coloniser is colonised: there is simply no time for the ordinary business of
  mundane day-to-day decision-making. In this way, the largely white, male
  governing oligarchy rely on and reproduce structures not only of gender
  but of class, ethnicity and age. Lifeworld detachment presupposes others'
  non-detachment.

Source: Adapted from Scambler (2013).

come together to form the governing oligarchy, are exclusive in their greed or
their instrumental use of others, far from it (Scambler, 2009). No more do they
exhaust the category of focused autonomous reflexives outlined here. *But* the
structuring of their internal conversations is pertinent to a sociology of health
inequalities that attributes due weight and attention to wealth and power as
well as to the simultaneous causal efficacy of structure and agency.

  These half-dozen attributes make up a plausible and sociologically useful
ideal-typical portrayal of the focused autonomous reflexive for a sociology of
health and health inequalities. A paragraph or two on ideology might back
this claim up. That people possess beliefs, values and attitudes, extending
even to dispositions, that owe more to their natal or involuntary placement

in society than to their exercise of agency 'seems as much an anachronism in sociology now as it was once a platitude' (Scambler, 2012b: 145). As much is central to Bhaskar's and Archer's realism, although each allows for the transformative power and potential of agency.

Unsurprisingly, those constituting the governing oligarchy are prime peddlers – via a mainstream media owned by billionaire tax exiles and think tanks explicitly funded to propagandise – of a neoliberal ideology that either applauds or excuses them. Recall Virchow and Engels's revolutionary opposition to the bourgeois ideologies of their day and place, vehicles of exploitation and oppression that helped undermine the health and longevity of the poor and powerless by strangling asset flows critical for their wellbeing: *ideology kills*. The role of the *symbolic*, indirect or circuitous as compared with overt, coercive, physical violence in producing and reproducing health inequalities has been neglected.

Vulnerable fractured reflexives

Wittgenstein (1958) again: where there exist the rich and powerful, there necessarily exist the poor and powerless. In postulating a subtype of Archer's fractured reflexives, the *vulnerable fractured reflexive*, I am implying neither more nor less than that there exist in contemporary Britain people who have learned what amounts to subservience. Archer (2012) argues that fractured reflexives have typically experienced severely disruptive life-events, lack longstanding solidary friendship networks and confidants, show dependency, lack notions of personal and work ambition and accomplishment and are passive in orientation. All this is consistent with my characterization of the vulnerable fractured reflexive sketched in Table 4.4.

The descriptor 'vulnerable' resonates with health and longevity. The vulnerable fractured reflexive, I maintain, is set up, although not of course predestined, for impaired health and wellbeing and a shortened life expectancy. I referred earlier to the relevance of a 'psychological asset flow' for health. Individuals can be demonstrably 'vulnerable' or 'resilient'; and it is obvious that these attributes are *in part* down to natal and social background and positioning, to 'involuntary placement' as well as to contingency and to happenstance *and therefore do not simply reduce to psychological precepts*. Agency, to reiterate, is structured but not structurally determined. As interactionists insist, 'who we (think we) are and how we evaluate ourselves impacts on our lives and our health' (Scambler, 2013: 311).

Building on this platform, I contend that vulnerable fractured reflexives comprise those most likely to be disadvantaged by the largely unintended consequences of the strategic action of the focused autonomous reflexives. A broadened umbrella concept of alienation is key. Yuill (2005)

Table 4.4 Attributes of the Vulnerable Fractured Reflexive

Lifeworld dependency
The vulnerable fractured reflexives (VFR) are sucked in and almost dry by the routines of the household or private sphere. The everyday tasks of 'getting by' (almost) ask too much.

Ships without anchor
The VFRs lack bearings, drifting, at the beck and call and mercy of Lyotard's (1971) 'petit narratives'. There is no core to who they are or why and what it all might amount to: it has been nibbled away by the cut and thrust of conditional circumstance.

Easily led
In need of rescue or guidance, they await the arrival of either the cavalry or an autonomous or meta-reflexive; but they await *without genuine hope or expectation*.

Open to ephemera
With no set compass and 'disoriented', they attach themselves to fads, fashions and the discourses of the moment, but without conviction; rather they are appendages or hangers on to the convictions and commitments of others.

Lacking personal projects
VFRs are characterised by 'passivity': they are Sartrean 'objects-for-others, underplaying any causal efficacy for want of personal aspiration or ambition.

Alienated
Expanding on Marx's classic exegesis, they are alienated in line with some or all of Seeman's (1959) dimensions: powerlessness, meaninglessness, normlessness, isolation and self-estrangement.

Of low self-worth and –esteem
Following on from their natal backgrounds and early life-events, impoverished sense of self, plus the 'self-fulfilling prophecy', they hold themselves of little account. Their outlook is informed by 'felt stigma' and/or 'felt deviance', a sense that they are either imperfect, inadequate or both.

Source: Adapted from Scambler (2013).

has rightly argued that the link between Marx's alienation and health has been neglected in health sociology; but Marx was writing 150 year ago. Moving on, I shall argue that the vulnerable fractured reflexives constitute an *absent presence* in the postmodern or relativised culture of financial capitalism. Vulnerable fractured reflexives, like those 'precariously' employed, can be found in all socioeconomic groups and classes. They live below the radar. Thus:

> to today's oligarchs they 'make up the numbers'. They are not floating voters in general elections: they may vote with tabloids like the 'Daily

Mail'; or, most likely, not at all. If they can be summed up in a phrase, then 'disconnected fatalists' might suffice. They are disconnected in an increasingly networked or connected world.

(Scambler, 2013: 312)

Disconnected fatalism is a socially structured subjectivity that predisposes to risk circumstances and behaviours for health and longevity.

While it may be that vulnerable fractured reflexives are prone to risk behaviours known to be injurious to health – smoking, excessive alcohol and fatty food consumption – and possibly also to the under-use of health and social services, this is not the whole story. Archer (2012) notes that they are liable to social immobility. My hypothesis is that they are they are less likely than others to be proactive, or even active, in contesting the strangulation or weakening of those asset flows known to be positive for health and longevity. If this is correct, then it follows that disadvantage emanating from involuntary placement and early childhood has a peculiar significance for this group.

'Life slips by.' An inherited firm goes bust under lackluster management; they forego opportunities for promotion or advancement, judging themselves fortunate to be in paid work at all; they did not buy their council house; the present recession is a 'fact of life'; universal credit represents a reasonable assessment of their worth.

(Scambler, 2013: 312)

There is more and deeper here than orthodox examinations of the social determinants of health and wellbeing and of shortened life expectancy. '*The part of the vulnerable fractured reflexives can only be grasped "against" the strategic behaviours of the focused autonomous reflexives. The former are in a sense the ongoing accomplishment of the latter*' (Scambler, 2013: 312–313). It does not follow of course that the strategic acts of the class-motivated governing oligarchy are the *sole* reason for the existence, attributes and lot of the vulnerable fractures reflexives, or that the circumstances of the latter can be *sufficiently* characterised as the by-product of class-based exploitation and command-based oppression. But I *am* claiming that exploitation and oppression are basic to their enduring disadvantage, that is, for any clustering and restriction of those asset flows salient for health and longevity.

Summing up at this point, I have sought to show something of the structuring of agency pertinent to a sociology of health inequalities. While the emphasis has been on focused autonomous and vulnerable fractured reflexives, signalling socially-induced advantageous and disadvantageous mind-sets or dispositions respectively, it is important to recognise the volatility of the causal input of these mind-sets or dispositions in what Bhaskar calls open systems. The causal powers of real structures or relations of class and command, and of structured agency too, considered as generative mechanisms issuing in tendencies, can be persuasive for a phenomenon like health inequalities in one context or figuration (e.g. Britain qua nation-state), and non-persuasive, annulled by other mechanisms (e.g. gender or ethnic relations), in another (e.g. a particular occupation or local community) (Scambler, 2002, 2005b).

Acts emanating from Britain's governing oligarchy might be reframed as risk behaviours for the health of others, perhaps most convincingly for vulnerable fractured reflexives. Is this too generous? Virchow and Engels, Marmot too, speak of 'killing'. Analyses of the prime owners of capital, in my terms Britain's capital executive comprising its monopolists, auxiliaries and 'sleepers' (see Chapter 3), and their ruthless instrumentality, lend credence to their accusations, and mine. Analyses of the backgrounds, interrelations and projects of the wealthy and powerful, and of the social structures they surf to their personal advantage, are conspicuous by the absence (an important concept in dialectical critical realism as we shall see in Chapter 5) in the sociology of health inequalities.

The focused autonomous reflexives are 'players' in the sociology of health inequalities, the vulnerable fractured reflexives 'non-players'. But another important qualification is in order. It is likely that reflexivity not only varies, or is capable of variation, per individual over time, but that it can vary too by status- and role-set. Merton maintained that each of us occupies a number (a set) of statuses (e.g. daughter, mother, school governor and so on), to each of which attaches a set of (role or) normative expectations (i.e. how appropriately to behave). Archer's modes of reflexivity might well vary – and enduringly so – by status- and role-set. This is a roundabout way of qualifying the applications here of Archer's conceptualization of reflexivity. Reflexivity almost certainly varies – systematically – by status- and its companion role-sets. This could explain why GBs raking in profits from casino-like betting on up-and-down exchange rates lovingly visit their grannies, walk their (pedigree) dogs with routine commitment and do unpaid stints in their local Oxfam bookshops through their early retirements *whilst cashing in on their capital investments*. The very same 'focused autonomous reflexives' whose uninhibited greed indirectly causes and fuels health inequalities may nevertheless be – and their characteristic cognitive dissonance may be relevant here – compliant communicative reflexives in the private sphere. When sociologists deploy ideal types, they are often accused of simplifying social reality; but those who charge them are, in turn, frequently charged with platitudinous and unhelpful references to and reminders of the 'complexity' of social reality. Not only can fairly settled modes of reflexivity change over the life-course, they can, arguably, vary by status- and role-set. We are each of us multiple personalities. What we *are* and *do* in one figuration, status- and role-set can and frequently does differ from what we *are* and *do* in another.

Some Mertonian middle-range theories

Thus far I have spelled out and elaborated on a single, if in my view the paramount, generative mechanism in financial capitalism. It is, I have argued, of singular importance for the sociology of health inequalities. But it can of course neither bear the whole weight of such a sociology nor exhaust it. I shall have more to say about this in subsequent chapters, but I conclude here by specifying four meso- or middle-range theories that help augment the discussion so far. Two are adaptations of the work of others, and two my own – although I suspect unoriginal – formulations.

Siegrist and 'effort/reward imbalance'

Siegrist (2009) has, after a longstanding programme of research, developed a theory or model purporting to contribute positively to our understanding and explanation of health inequalities. His core tenet is that when people put in a sustained effort, either in their paid employment or in extra-work activities, *and their commitment is un- or under-appreciated,* then this impacts negatively on their health. It is a theory in close alliance with Marmot's research on the health costs of lack of work autonomy and on the relevance for health of 'status syndrome'. Articulating Siegrist's model in the context of my advocacy of the class/command dynamic as *the* dominant generative mechanism of financial capitalism, and of the GBH, I would suggest that it affords a meso-social, mediatory or contributory mechanism to a comprehensive sociological explanation of enduring health inequalities by helping account for the diminished health of people struggling on zero hours contracts, benefit cuts and so on. Felt stigma and deviance can wound and kill.

Goldthorpe and 'relative risk aversion'

Goldthorpe, whose latest book places him much closer, quantitatively if not qualitatively, to critical realism than he might care to admit (Goldthorpe, 2016), came up with a 'relative risk aversion' model to account for the non-fluid character of social mobility in Britain. This model asserted that:

> when making educational choices with their futures in mind, young people, and their parents, will give priority to the avoidance of downward social mobility over the achievement of upward mobility. However, while risk aversion can then be seen as equal, relative to social origins, 'the actual risks involved' in educational choice will be unequal. For children of more advantaged social origins, there will be little to lose, in seeking to maintain their parents' position, by taking up all further educational opportunities that their previous performance makes available to them – and even if their chances of ultimate success may be doubtful. But for children of less advantaged social origins, educational choice will be more problematic. For,

in their case, more ambitious choices that might end in failure could not only be in various ways costly in themselves but could also preclude less ambitious choices that, even if not offering great prospects for advancement, would at all events still effectively guard against downward mobility. Consequently, for these children to make a more ambitious choice, they would need to have a greater assurance of success – as would be indicated by a higher level of previous performance – than would their more advantaged counterparts.

(Goldthorpe, 2016: 118–119)

I want to suggest that this model has applicability too in the health domain. A propensity to 'play safe' adversely affects the health and longevity of those – often natally – disadvantaged, and especially vulnerable fractured reflexives, more than it does those more advantageously placed. It is a model that mitigates against tansformatory action.

Ego adjustment

I am concerned here with a social rather than a psychological mechanism and one that shapes people's definitions of their situations. It is a middle-range model asserting that people's definitions of self, situation and orientation to social change mirror the Mertonian status- and role-sets they occupy. This applies not only to their natal placement but to the dynamics of any social mobility. In other words, people 'rationalise' their definitions to fit their circumstances. The empirically-ratified 'logic' here is that those born to advantage, *plus* the minority who are upwardly mobile, *adjust* their conceptions of the good society to coincide with, 'fit' and justify their pecuniary and other interests. The relevance to health and health care is obvious. Boldly expressed, as people's material (and associated) asset flows strengthen, so does their willingness to attribute personal responsibility for 'lifestyle decision-making' to those less advantaged and to tolerate, consider and ultimately vote for measures to privatise the NHS and, further down the line, to take out personal health insurance.

Activity reinforcement

What becomes familiar matters more, more insistently structures agency and is more causally efficacious than is often appreciated. While Bourdieu was right to emphasise the salience of a class-based habitus, there exist a myriad of other stable or settled predispositions to action. The notion of an epilepsy habitus was pressed into service earlier. The activity reinforcement model here points to a tendency for the repetition-cum-familiarity associated with status- and role-set occupancy to translate into a behavioural predictability beyond the conscious reach of ego adjustment. It becomes 'natural' to settle into an atomistic individualism intrinsic to financial capitalism's neoliberal ideology of capital accumulation when one's material asset flow reaches a turning point (which assists focused autonomous reflexivity). In similar vein, it becomes natural too for those with more meagre asset flows whose lives tilt towards disconnected fatalism to 'know their lot', however resentfully (which assists vulnerable fractured reflexivity). Adherence to a low/high rates of inheritance tax is positively associated with the amount people aspire to pass on.

To pull together the threads of this chapter, agency is structured but never structurally determined; and as Archer has convincingly argued, we take off from our natal circumstances and our first and secondary socialisation to ease our way into an agency that holds out a variable potential for social transformation. Reflexivity typically (that is, more often than not), and here each of the four middle-range theories or models adumbrated above comes into play, shifts subtly to coincide with financial capitalism's primary generative mechanism, the class/command dynamic, whilst also – to recollect critical realism's stance on open systems – remaining responsive by status- and role-sets, figuration-by-figuration and level-by-level to other mechanisms. Social life is emergent, complex or messy.

How do these paragraphs on socially structured agency and reflexivity knit in with my overall thesis on the social maldistribution of health and longevity? In previous published and blogged accounts, the emphasis has been on restoring and highlighting the neglected role of social structures in general, and of relations of class and command in particular, in the sociology of health inequalities. Sociologists have too often adopted the agenda, entirely legitimate in its own right *but not as a proxy for doing sociology*, of social epidemiologists; and in the process, they have routinely subsumed explanation in prediction (see the discussion of positivism in Chapter 2). As outlined in Chapter 3, the hard core of my thesis is that the principal structural mechanism of financial capitalism is its revised class/command dynamic. How this mechanism plays out in the transnational, national, regional and local patterning of the 'events' that we observe and monitor is of course variable; but it is my contention that it dwarfs other mechanisms active at the level or figuration of the nation state as the prepotent cause of health inequalities. The strategic behaviour of members of Britain's capitalist executive, and most conspicuously its monopolists, constitutes a pathological risk factor for sickness and premature demise, most especially amongst those 'precariously' located on the periphery of the working class.

The most notable media of enactment of the class/command dynamic are the set of asset flows outlined in the previous chapter, considered not only objectively but also subjectively (i.e. in the light of people's own definitions of their situation in terms of the strength of their asset flows relative to those of others in their reference groups). In this way, neo-Marxist conflict theory draws on the insights of symbolic interactionism. I hope to show later that the four middle-range or meso-theories outlined, retroductively or abductively inferable mechanisms in their own right, help account for the causal impact of the class/command dynamic on the maldistribution of morbidity and mortality.

While Bhaskar's transformational model has been sympathetically articulated, and the existence and potential of agency affirmed throughout, there remains a lot more to be said. Archer's contribution has been to show how those internal conversations we hold so dear are: (a) real, and forces for change, and (b) mediated by structure and context. In the next chapter, the brief will be to further complicate the sociological examination of health and life-expectancy by dipping wary toes into the deep and murky waters of Bhaskar's dialectical critical realism, and in even more peremptory fashion into his Meta-Reality.

5 The sociological potential of dialectical critical realism

Thus far reference and use have been restricted to what Bhaskar came to call basic critical realism. In this chapter I introduce elements of his *dialectical critical realism* (DCR) (Bhaskar, 1993). His dialectical arguments, I shall maintain, are worth visiting despite their somewhat arcane, philosophical dexterity. I open the chapter by tracing the evolution of this stage of his evolving project in sufficient detail as to render intelligible my own modest later use of it. Apart from Bhaskar himself, I draw liberally on the sympathetic but critical study of Creaven (2007), who argues for a Marxist adaptation of DCR, and, less so, on the more straightforward account of Norrie (2010), a philosopher of law and friend and accomplice of Bhaskar.

The core of dialectical critical realism

Bhaskar positions his analysis within the dialectical tradition of Hegel and Marx. His aim is to deepen his basic critical realism by developing a general theory of dialectic sufficiently robust to underwrite a meta-theory of the social sciences that would release them to function as agencies of human emancipation. He aspired to provide, in his own words, 'a philosophical basis for Marxian social theory consistent with Marx's own undeveloped methodological insights'. This requires the philosophical under-labouring for a genuinely emancipatory socialist political project.

Bhaskar started by critiquing Hegel's notion of the dialectic. The problem with Hegel's logic, he averred, is that it eradicates the dualisms of thought and reality and of subject and object en route to a complete and self-consistent idealism. Dialectic for Hegel is a logical process of the re-unification of opposites, transcendence of limitations and reconciliation of differences. Bhaskar warrants quoting at some length here:

> From the vantage point of (positive) reason the mutual exclusivity of opposites passes over into the recognition of their reciprocal interdependence (mutual inclusion): they remain inseparable yet distinct moments in a richer, more total conceptual formation (which will in turn generate a new contradiction of its own). It is the constellational identity of

understanding and reason within reason which fashions the continually recursively expanding kaleidoscopic tableaux of absolute idealism ... Dialectic ... is ... the process by which the various categories, notions or forms of consciousness arise out of each other to inform ever more inclusive totalities until the system of categories, notions or forms as a whole is completed.

(Bhaskar, 1993: 581)

Enlightenment amounts to a process of *negating negation*. It culminates in the 'achieved constellational identity' of subject and object in consciousness 'as thought finally grasps the world as a rational totality, *as part of itself*, which exists as rational totality in order to enable philosophical self-consciousness to be achieved.' The unification of subject and object, then, is the process by which reason (or better, Reason) becomes self-conscious. This is the *telos* of the Hegelian system, the historical moment when totality becomes 'constellationally' closed or completed (Creaven, 2007: 21).

So, setting aside its removal from Anglo-Saxon thinking (at least since the early decades of the last century), what according to Bhaskar is wrong with Hegel's ambitious, all-encompassing or absolute idealism? It is clearly at odds with his basic critical realist philosophy: most obviously, it bulldozes over the ontological reality of stratification and emergence. Bhaskar seeks to show that the realist notions of stratification and emergence cannot lend themselves to Hegel's idea of a closed totality; thus undermining the latter's 'identity' of subjective and objective dialectics. For Bhaskar, good totalities are open, bad totalities are closed.

The non-identity of subject and object, Bhaskar argues, ensures that there is no reason why all being must be 'conceivable' being, let alone why all being must be conceived of already. The fact that the cosmos is an 'open totality' ensures that there is always the possibility, or likelihood, of newly emergent strata – crucially for us in this volume, the possibility of new social structures brought about by human agency – so that reality is forever incomplete and inherently impossible to grasp fully.

This interpretation by Bhaskar supports the *unity-in-difference* of being and consciousness that is at the core of materialistic dialectics. Creaven (2007: 21) again:

> For Bhaskar, because strata are 'equal members of the same hierarchy, (they have) an aspect of unity (dualism or pluralism is rejected)'; at the same time, because 'the strata are not the same as, nor reducible to, one another ... they have an aspect of difference (reductionism is rejected)'.

What Bhaskar calls Hegel's 'cognitive triumphalism' reduces the world to a non-hierarchical flat space with fixed boundaries and dimensions, arresting the ongoing process of determinate negation in physical and social systems alike. This denies the existence of 'multiple totalities' and of the openness and incompleteness of each of these. This can of course lead to the 'epistemic fallacy': questions about the world collapse into questions about what we can/do know about the world (ontology is reduced to epistemology).

So Hegel's dialectic fails to meet Bhaskar's criteria. It is also, he maintains, internally flawed. If, as Hegel insists, truth consists in totality and the conformity of an object to its notion, then he *ought* to accept that the idea of an open totality is more true – that is, complete and adequate – than the idea of a closed totality; after all, it is more comprehensive and encompassing and 'contains the latter as a special case'. Creaven (2007: 22) summarises:

> Logically, the structures of reality have to be grasped as 'open-ended', if Hegel's 'progressivist' conceptualization of dialectic as the movement towards a richer, fuller, more universal consciousness is to be upheld.

Bhaskar will have no truck with the triadic process of negation generally associated with Hegel (thesis-antithesis-synthesis). Dialectics for him is not simply about a putative law of the interpenetration of opposites in a given structure or system, leading to their 'preservative sublation' in a new structure or system (a higher totality). Dialectical processes, Bhaskar insists, are not always sublatory (or supersessive), let alone preservative; nor are they always characterised by opposition or antagonism. On the contrary, many are characterised by 'mere connection, separation or juxtaposition'.

In the most general of terms, Bhaskar defines dialectic as 'any kind of interplay between differentiated but related elements'. More specifically, he sees dialectic 'as structure-in-process and process-in-structure by virtue of the interconnections and oppositions which bring about the elaboration or transformation of a given system or totality or of some or more of its elements'. In his own words, dialectical thinking is 'the art of thinking the *coincidence of distinctions and connections.*'

Hegel came to privilege unity over difference. Bhaskar reverses this. It is timely here to recall a tenet or two of basic critical realism. Each (ontological) stratum can be conceptualised in isolation from any concept in the stratum from which it is emergent or in which it is rooted (the champion is necessarily emergent from/rooted in them, but cells don't win Wimbledon). It follows that 'in *reality* there is nothing *present* in the emergent stratum connecting it to the root stratum. Because of this ... it is the aspect of difference that requires emphasis within the critical realist ontology' (Brown, 2002: 173).

If for Hegel the dialectical process denotes the logic of negation, Bhaskar emphasises 'negative dialectics' as (generally) the absenting of absence and (specifically) 'the absenting of constraints on absenting absences or ills' (hopefully this will become a little clear later on). Although he distinguishes between conceptual, social and natural dialectical processes, he regards all of these as 'energized by the logic of absence or negation'. Creaven (2007: 23) again:

Ontologically, the process is synonymous with social and natural geo-history. Epistemologically, the process is synonymous with progress in philosophical and theoretical thought, particularly the logic of scientific discovery. Normatively-practically, the process is precisely 'the axiology of freedom'.

In a bid to 'radicalise' Hegel, Bhaskar defines the core dialectical category as 'real determinate absence or non-being'. Negativity here becomes 'the lynchpin of all dialectics'. This negativity or absence is not simply a property of (the incompleteness of) conceptual thought, *but of the ontological status of reality itself.* This is crucial. Bhaskar argues against what he terms 'ontological monovalence', or a 'purely positive, complementing a purely actual, notion of reality'. He insists rather on the necessity of absence or non-being – that is, on 'negative dialectics' – given the open-ended nature of reality.

> If negativity or absence were entirely cancelled out by positive being, the dialectic would cease, and with it change, development, evolution, emergence, leaving us with Hegel's 'constellationally' closed totality ('endism').
>
> (Creaven, 2007: 23)

Hegel's 'absenting of the notion of absence' betrays the positivity of absolute idealism. Creaven (2007: 24) continues:

> For Hegel there was history, but in capitalist modernity there is no longer. Positive being reigns supreme. Argues Bhaskar, 'the chief result of ontological monovalence in mainstream philosophy is to erase the contingency of existential questions and to despatialise and detemporalise being'.

Negativity, for Bhaskar, is a condition of positive being; and so absence or non-being is ontologically prior to presence or being. *Absence or non-being is an ocean, presence or being merely a ripple on its surface.* 'Real determinate absence or negativity energizes the struggle for presence or positivity. This is the essence of dialectic' (Creaven, 2007: 24).

Bhaskar's explication of negativity provides the basis for his analysis of *contradiction*. His definition of contradiction is a broad one: it can be taken, he suggests, as a kind of metaphor to cover 'any kind of dissonance, strain or tension'. But there are discernible types of contradiction. At root, contradiction 'specifies a situation which permits the satisfaction of one end or more generally results only at the expense of another; that is, a bind or constraint'. An *internal contradiction* occurs when there is a double bind or self-constraint (which may be multiplied to form a knot):

In this case a system, agent or structure, S, is blocked from performing with one system, rule or principle, R, because it is performing with another, R1; or, a course of action, T, generates a countervailing, inhibiting, T1. R1 and T1 are radically negating of R and T respectively.

(Creaven, 2007: 25)

Internal contradictions are essential to the possibility of emergent entities and of change as a self-implementing process.

The notion of *external contradiction* refers to laws and constraints of nature – like the speed of light – to be established by the mere fact of determinate spatiotemporal being. The notion embraces the limiting conditions or binds imposed on humans and societies by force of natural necessity. Creaven (2007: 25) extrapolates:

> In terms of society, the concept may perhaps also usefully refer to the inter-relations that exist between structures of a given system or social formation, insofar as these are not relations of mutual presupposition (i.e. internal and necessary connections between elements of an institutional whole), but insofar as these entail mutual incompatibilities or strains between elements of the total system. But, in fact, these can be said to be simultaneously external and intrinsic contradictions: 'intrinsic' insofar as these are strains or incompatibilities between the constitutive structures of a unitary social system (e.g. those between capitalism and liberalism's own legal and political norms of 'justice' and 'democracy'); 'external' insofar as each constituent structure of a social system (economic, political, religious, educational etc) is constituted and defined by a specific configuration of roles, rules, norms and positions, which are mutually antagonistic.

Formal logical contradiction is a form of internal contradiction 'whose consequences for the subject, unless the terms of redescribed and/or the discursive domain is expanded ... is axiological indeterminacy' (i.e. the lack of rational grounds for action).

The notion of dialectical contradiction is another form of internal contradiction. These can be radical or transformative depending on whether they negate 'the source of the existential incompatibility between elements of the totality or the common ground of the totality itself', or whether they inform 'processes of dynamic restructuring which can be contained within a given totality or which do not sublate its common ground'.

Gradually, via this synopsis of Bhaskar on contradiction in particular, a link with Marx and a potential salience for substantive sociology is revealed. Bhaskar has gone beyond (his reading of) Hegel and given ontological anchorage to the concept of dialectic. Bhaskar agrees with much of what Marx has to say about Hegel. Crucially, Marx's materialist dialectics, unlike Hegel's idealistic dialectics, does *not* dissolve objective dialectical contradictions into subjective logical contradictions. Materialistic dialectical contradictions such as those identified by Marx *describe (dialectical), but do not suffer from (logical) contradictions*. Creaven (2007: 26) summarises:

> the practical resolution of the contradiction here is the non-preservative transformative negation of the ground of the internally relational but 'tendentially mutually exclusive' totality of which they are a part, this requiring the intervention of practical human agency in the social and material worlds.

In Bhaskar's view, Marx's critique of Hegel opens up the possibility of a 'materialist diffraction of dialectic': that is, 'the articulation of a pluriform dialectic, enfolding at various levels of conceptual thought and objective reality' (Creaven, 2007: 27). According to Bhaskar, what he terms the 'four levels' of DCR are perhaps best seen as four dimensions of this diffracted dialectic, each with its own distinctive concepts, scientific applications and philosophical problems.

Unsurprisingly, Bhaskar's 'pluriform' dialectic is more complex than anything to be found in Marx or in his disciples and interpreters. Creaven usefully offers an example of (unreconstructed) Marxian dialectics at work. Consider, he says, Marx and Engels's 'dialectic of labour'. There is more than an echo of Hegel here. On the one hand, Marx contends that the relationship between humans and their environment must be seen as a contradictory totality, a unity of opposites:

> The unity is derived from the fact that nature is the 'inorganic body' of human thought and action, with which human beings 'must remain in continual interchange' if they 'are not to die', humanity being 'a part of nature.' The opposition is derived from the fact that, although human consciousness is a product of nature, it is nonetheless a qualitatively distinct part of nature, by virtue of its power to reflect upon and transform nature in the service of human needs, and because it must still encounter the world as an objective power, as a set of circumstances which confront and constrain thought and action from without.
>
> (Creaven, 2007: 27)

On the other hand, this contradictory totality, which constitutes the relationship between human subjects and objective conditions, is a dynamic and developing one. This is the case because collaborative labour on the material world that is oriented to human subjects' needs and interests 'mediates the two poles', drawing thought into a closer correspondence with its objects, 'combining materiality and consciousness as conscious "practice"', and in the process, transcending, 'without harmonizing', the 'abstract polarities represented by both sides of this existential contradiction' (Creaven, 2007: 27).

So what does Bhaskar add (and does it warrant all this arduous mental labour)? In his *Dialectic: the Pulse of Freedom*, he claims that his philosophical under-labouring is indispensable to Marxian social theory and emancipatory socialist politics. So, now we return to his four levels of DCR.

Bhaskar reworked Hegel's dialectic via the concepts of non-identity, negativity, totality and transformative agency. These four concepts are mapped onto his four levels of DCR. What he dubs the *first moment* (1M) can be seen as corresponding to the core notions of basic critical realism (e.g. stratification, emergence, the non-identity of thought and being, system openness and so on).

The *second edge* (2E) 'is the abode of absence – and, most generally, negativity'. This involves a 'remodelling' of the core notions of 1M in the light of dialectical categories such as negativity, negation, becoming, contradiction, process, development and decline, mediation and reciprocity. 2E imparts dynamism to basic critical realism, allowing for processes of change to be situated spatially and temporally.

The *third level* (3L) corresponds to totality (and 'totalising motifs'). Bhaskar maintains that the 'internal and intrinsic connectedness of phenomena' deducible from the 'dialecticisation' of 1M at 2E reveals the need for totalising motifs that can theorise totality and constellationality.

This gives rise to the *fourth dimension* (4D): this is 'the zone of transformative agency', the unity of theory and practice *in practice*. This is

> the process of human practical engagement with the world, in society and nature, which also mediates the poles of consciousness and being, bringing thought into a 'lived relation' with the world, thereby transcending (though without harmonizing) the abstract polarities represented by subject and object.
>
> (Creaven, 2007: 29)

Bhaskar counters extant 'erroneous' interpretations of this 'zone' (e.g. physicalism, idealism, dualism, reification, fetishism, commodification). He also offers the conceptual means of their resolution, which hinges on synchronous emergent powers materialism at the level of subject and the dialectic of structure and agency at the level of society.

The interface of 3L and 4D can also be presented as the 'moment' of 'dialectical critical naturalism', or the theorization of society as unity-in-difference, and maps onto Bhaskar's transformational model of social action. This is, or at least ought to be in my view, of special interest to sociologists. Creaven (2007: 29) writes:

> According to Bhaskar's transformational model of social action, social forms (institutions, roles, positions, belief-systems, etc) are legitimate objects of scientific knowledge, because they are autonomous of the human agents that reproduce them through their activity, and because

they possess their own causal efficacy. These properties (autonomy and causality) secure the objects of the social sciences as 'real'. This autonomy of social forms does not consist of activity-independence, but rather of their 'anteriority' or pre-existence to any specific passage of human interaction across time and space.

It will be remembered that for Bhaskar, human agents do not create society, but always find it ready-made: they reproduce or transform it through their interaction. This is important enough to warrant the repetition of a summative point made earlier:

> Society is both the ever-present condition (material cause) and the continually reproduced outcome of human agency ... Society ... provides necessary conditions for intentional human action, and intentional human action is a necessary condition for it. Society is only present in human action, but human action always expresses and utilizes some or other social form ... People do not create society. For it always pre-exists them and is a necessary condition for their activity. Rather, society must be regarded as an ensemble of structures, practices and conventions which individuals reproduce or transform, but which would not exist unless they did so. Society does not exist independently of human activity (the error of reification). But it is not the product of it (the error of voluntarism).
>
> (Bhaskar, 1998: 34–35)

Social structures are conceived here as 'enabling', not just constraining or coercive. They are not reducible to their effects, *but they only present through them*. For Bhaskar, the transformational model of social action outperforms, sees off, the individualism of Weber, the collectivism of Durkheim and the phenomenology of Berger. The transformational model of social action goes hand in hand with a *relational* – rather than individualist, collectivist or interactionist – conception of society. So sociologists are charged with investigating social order as a 'position-practice system'.

Bhaskar wants via DCR to 'generalize, dialecticise and substantialise the transformational model of social action'. He wants to incorporate the complexities of power and conflict. He is in pursuit, it might be said, of DCR as sociology, politics and ethics.

He (Bhaskar & Norrie, 1998: 566) offers what he describes as a 'naturalistically-grounded four planar' theory of the possibilities of social being:

> Social life, qua totality, is constituted by four dialectically interdependent planes: of material transactions with nature, inter-personal action, social relations, and intra-subjectivity.

This four planar theory leads him to write of 'the social cube', a complex multi-dimensional articulation of ensembles of structure-practice-subject in process. How does this complement and add to his transformational model of social action? It will be recalled that the original version emphasised that social structure is a necessary condition for, and medium of, intentional agency, which is in turn a necessary condition for the reproduction or transformation of social forms. Creaven (2007: 31) summarises its limitations as follows:

> The difficulty with this model is that it is rather too abstract or generalizing to offer much theoretical purchase on the complexity of structural conditioning and the problem of the construction of human material as subjects, actors and agents of social reproduction/transformation.

What the four planar model recognises, and allows for, is that these processes occur on a number of interlinked levels of terrains. To clarify:

> For Bhaskar, it is the dialectical interaction of agents with structural properties and/or practices on these analytically distinct planes (material transactions with nature, i.e. co-operative labour to produce subsistence; social relations between agents, i.e. as incumbents of structured 'positions' and 'practices' of the social system; interpersonal relations, i.e. interactions between individuals as subjects rather than as agents of positions or institutional roles; and intra-subjective relations, i.e. internal relations of the subject, such as the self-construction of personal and cultural identities), which constitute the social cube.
>
> (Creaven, 2007: 31)

Bhaskar again: '*we have dialectics of unity and diversity, of intrinsic and extrinsic, of part and whole, of centrification and peripheralisation, within partial totalities in complex and dislocated open process, substantively under the configuration of global commodification*' (Bhaskar, 1998: 645).

As with society, individuals are in this revised transformational model of social action presented as stratified and relational entities, 'as existentially constituted by their rhythmics or geo-histories and the totality of their relations with other things' (Bhaskar, 1993: 62). At this point, a distinction between 'power 1' and 'power 2' becomes relevant. Power 1 relations refer straightforwardly to 'the transformative capacity intrinsic to the concept of agency as such'. Power 2 encompasses a more sociological notion of power. Power 2, recalling C Wright Mills's analysis, denotes social relations that govern the distribution of material goods, political and military authority and social and cultural stratification. Power 2 relations are those that enable agents to defend their sectoral advantages by prevailing against either the covert wishes and/or the real interests of others. Bhaskar wants to emphasise here that power is enabling/empowering as well as repressive.

> The significance of power2 relations, argues Bhaskar, is not that they grant agents the capacity to exercise control over the social and natural

environments, the capacity to intervene causally in the world, which is an unqualified good, but that they organize or structure an uneven distribution of the capacity of human agents to exercise transformative power over their conditions of existence, and so restrict the autonomy and free-flourishing of people subject to their governance.

(Creaven: 2007: 32)

Also salient here is Bhaskar's political-moral theory, in which 'concrete singularity' (or the free-flourishing of *each*) is the relational condition of 'concrete universality' (or the free-flourishing of *all*). He sees this as 'an imminent and tendential possibility ... necessitated by structural conditions ... (though) held in check by global discursively moralized power 2 relations'. He announces a (contingent) progressive tendential movement of humanity towards 'eudaimonia', or universal emancipation.

How to make this clearer? We must return to Bhaskar's definition of dialectic as the process of 'absenting absence'. Dialectic entails 'absenting most notably of constraints on desires, wants, needs and interests'. In a sentence, the dialectic of freedom is powered by the interface of absence and desire, since absence is paradigmatically a condition for desire (since desire presupposes lack). Humanity, Bhaskar maintains, is bestowed with the 'inner urge' to struggle against lack 'that flows universally from the logic of elemental ... need, want'; and this is manifested 'wherever power2 relations hold sway'. This is because power 2 relations negate the needs, ranging from those of basic survival to those defined by culture, of most humans, leading to a desire for freedom from 'absenting ills'. Creaven (2007: 33) elaborates:

> This marks a welcome departure from the 'mutual constitution' model of structure-agency linkages of the original transformational model of social action, whereby structures govern all intentional acts of human beings. This is because it is clear here that Bhaskar wishes to invoke the enduring needs and interests of human nature to naturalistically ground resistance to those social relations that would deny or curtail or limit those needs or interests. It is this process of struggle against absence or lack that offers the tendential possibility or even geo-political impulse of moving 'from primal scream to universal human emancipation'. Since 'every absence can be seen as a constraint, this goal of human autonomy can be regarded as implicit in the infant's primal scream'.

The unfolding dialectic of absenting absence on freedom – as agents struggle against successive forms of power 2 relations – taken together with expanding cultural definitions of needs and wants constructed in part through this struggle, nurtures and fuels a logic of more inclusive and encompassing definitions of and aspirations towards freedom.

Although he characterises the dialectic of freedom as a process of acting to absent constraining ills, Bhaskar does not draw the line at what Creaven calls 'practical agency energised by material interests'. Rather he extends the analysis to embrace communicative action more generally, including moral or ethical judgements:

> Insofar as an ill is unwanted, unneeded and remedial, the spatio-temperal-causal-absenting or real transformative negation of the ill presupposes universalizability to absenting agency in all dialectically similar circumstances. This presupposes in turn the absenting of all similar constraints. And by the inexorable logic of dialectical universalizability, insofar as all constraints are similar in virtue of 'their being constraints', i.e. qua constraints, this presupposes the absenting of all constraints as such ... And this presupposes in its wake a society oriented to the free development and flourishing of each and all, and of each as a condition for all, that is to say, universal autonomy as flourishing ... So the goal of universal human autonomy is implicit in every moral judgement.
>
> (Bhaskar, 1993: 263–264)

So, for Bhaskar, to act is to absent is to presuppose universal human emancipation. This adds up to a dialectic of universalization in practical and ethical interests. In recognizing and acting to negate the constraining ills that threaten their own 'concrete singularity', actors are committed to recognizing and acting to negate the constraining ills that threaten others who share common situations and a common human-social-being-in-nature ('concrete universality'). In this way, Bhaskar 'naturalistically grounds his moral realism and ethical naturalism in a four-planar theory of changing and changeable human nature-in-nature', by virtue of which human interactions objectively presuppose trust, solidarity and mutual aid. (Creaven, 2007: 34). Not that this makes the future predictable. At the beginning of Bhaskar's dialectic is non-identity, at the end open, unfinished totality, along with the unity-in-difference of consciousness and being.

DCR, health and health inequalities

The preceding paragraphs have necessarily comprised a lengthy, though in fact abbreviated, dense and tough-reading sub-section for those unfamiliar with Bhaskar's writings. Can this be justified? I will argue that it can in a variety of respects, starting with a discussion of its potentials and going on to list ways in which it might facilitate conceptual and theoretical innovation in sociology generally and the sociology of health and health inequalities in particular. In the remainder of this chapter, the focus is largely on: (a) professional, policy and critical sociologies, to be extended in Chapter 6; and (b) public, foresight and action sociologies, to be extended in Chapter 8 (see also Chapter 2).

Diagnostic dialectics

The concepts of absence and negation have been situated within DCR in the preceding paragraphs. Understood as an ocean of non-being upon which being occasionally causes a ripple or two, absence is the hinge that permits much else. It can take many forms. Perhaps most conspicuously it reminds us of Schutz's challenge to the 'natural attitude' (see Chapter 2). For all that we tend to assume that the socially structured world we inhabit constitutes some kind of ineluctable conclusion or climax to the past, this bears interrogation.

Paraphrasing Derrida, Badiou (2016: 130) illustrates *both* the substantive *and* the emancipatory potential of grasping the salience of absence:

> In Marx's analysis of bourgeois or capitalist societies, the proletariat is truly the non-existent characteristic of political municipal multiplicities. It is 'that which does not exist'. That does not mean that it has no being by any means. Marx does not think for a moment that the proletariat has no being, as he will, on the contrary, write volume after volume to explain what it is. The social and economic being of the proletariat is not in doubt. What is in doubt, always has been, and is now so more than ever, is its political 'existence'. The proletariat is that which has been completely removed from political representation. The multiplicity that it is can be analysed but, if we take the rules of appearance in the political world, it does not appear there. It is there, but with a minimal degree of appearance, or in other words a degree zero of appearance. That is obviously what the 'Internationale' sings: 'We are nothing, let us be all.' What does 'we are nothing' mean? Those who proclaim 'we are nothing' are not asserting their nothingness. They are simply stating that they are nothing in the world as it is, when it comes to appearing politically. From the point of view of their political appearance, they are nothing. And becoming 'all' presupposes a change of world, or in other words a change of transcendental. The transcedental must change the ascription of an existence, and therefore a non-existence or the point of a multiplicity's non-appearance in a world, is to change in its turn.

'Absence teaches us different and difference, opens up alternate 'possible worlds': *what is need not be.* An acknowledgement of (the ocean of) absence or non-being exposes our (ripple of a) positive world as a system open for transformation' (Scambler & Scambler, 2015: 349). Achieving transformation, or 'structural elaboration' in Archer's vocabulary, is another matter, as we shall see. Absence, Bhaskar (2016: 119–120) contends, has considerable 'diagnostic value': 'looking at a social situation and asking what is *not* there, what is missing, will often give the researcher an invaluable insight into how the situation needs to change and/or how it will change.'

Scambler and Scambler (2015: 349–351) consider the professional and policy literature on 'tackling health inequalities' in light of the notion of absence. They cite in particular the report of the WHO (2008) *Commission on Social Determinants of Health*. Documentation in this report noted a gap in life expectancy at birth of 40 years between affluent and non-affluent societies. Gross inequalities in health status were found to divide echelons within all countries. The Commission's recommendations covered three fields: (a) improving daily living conditions; (b) tackling the inequitable distribution of power, money and resources; and (c) studying and evaluating both the problem and the impact of interventions.

It may seem strange on the face of it to associate, let alone confront, such recommendations with charges of absence. After all, they appear to prescribe precisely the measures commended. At one level, that of Burawoy's (2005) 'policy sociology', they are indeed apt, subtle and hard-hitting. Moreover, Marmot's counsel might appropriately be characterised as diplomatic and compelling: his WHO report was, to recall Habermas, strategically constructed to co-opt pragmatic governance. But a price was paid: it glosses over the contradictions of capitalism. Bhaskar's notion of the 'real' disappears into the ether. Commenting on this, coupled with Marmot's (2010) UK report on health inequalities, Scambler and Scambler (2015: 349) write:

> in skating over capitalism's multiple contradictions the reports effectively underwrite a class ideology reflective of the vested interests of the capitalist-executive-oriented power elite (and their coterie of advisers and hangers-on within the new middle class).

Coburn's (2009: 44) uncompromising statement warrants a re-quote here (see Chapter 3):

> People with high SES (socio-economic status) do indeed live longer than those with less. SES, however, is a mere ranking of people according to income, educational attainment or occupational position. It reflects standards of living generally, and because these standards are related to many different types of disease, it is a good correlate of health status. But SES is itself the outcome of class forces. The nature of the capitalist class structure, and the outcome of class struggles, determine the extent and type of socio-economic inequalities in a given society, and the socio-economic inequalities in turn shape the pattern of health – and of health care. But while many theorists of the social determinants of health proclaim an interest in the basic determinants of health and health inequalities, much of their literature omits any consideration whatsoever of the political and class causes of SES and the SES-health relationship. When they speak of analysing the 'causes' of disease, they seldom go far enough up the causal chain to confront the class forces and class struggles that are ultimately determinant.

Absent from the WHO and many another socio-epidemiological/policy sociological report, in short, is any account of the deep, underlying generative mechanisms accessible via retroductive or abductive inference that speak only too eloquently of the causal efficacy of class and command.

> The price paid for what is a thoroughly dubious – because it is the very antithesis of 'evidence-based' – aspiration for reform is the failure to get to grips with, *to misrepresent*, capitalism and its contradictions, and a consequent suppression of the case for a more revolutionary rethink.
>
> (Scambler & Scambler, 2013: 92)

Absence offers more. Those comprising the governing oligarchy are no less absent from the sociology of health inequalities, notwithstanding their role as enforcers of the class/command dynamic. In fact, the contemporary, 'taming' fixation on population-wide indices of socioeconomic group or status, feeble proxies for social class, precludes analyses of the governing oligarchy, its invisible presence within their various premier categories amounting to absence. This cannot be dismissed as coincidental but is instead an indirect product of power 2 relations (Scambler, 1996).

Power 1 relations proclaim agency's causal proclivity to transform. Power 2 relations announce a desire to negate constraining ills. The neo-Marxist approach to the sociology of health inequalities defended here lends itself to a neophyte theory of power 2 relations pertaining to health and longevity. Health inequalities can only be explained sociologically by drawing on the real generative mechanism of class and, as Bhaskar affirms, class *struggle*.

> In financial capitalism it is the hardened core or cabal within Britain's increasingly finance-oriented transnational capitalist executive that commandeers the state's power elite to deliver its agenda, and a by-product of this agenda is a staggering boost to wealth, income and, in its wake, health inequality. It is Britain's governing oligarchy that most notably occasions, reproduces, underwrites and in today's financial capitalism intensifies its health inequalities.
>
> (Scambler & Scambler, 2015: 351)

But absence has purchase beyond sociological explanation or diagnostics. It can inform sociology beyond its professional, policy and critical guises. In Chapter 2, I re-rehearsed an argument advanced initially 20 year ago, one that developed Habermas's (1984) notion of lifeworld rationalisation (Scambler, 1996). My contention was that sociology is necessarily part and parcel of a reconstructed (most notably, post-foundationalist) or neo-Enlightenment 'project of modernity': in other words, sociology is *logically* and *morally* at one with lifeworld rationalisation (see also Chapter 8). It *has* to be pitted against *any* ideology that comes between it and its accounts of how social phenomena are and why. For Bhaskar, this is part of an

emancipatory project rooted in contesting those power 2 relations, constituting constraining ills, that deprive *most* humans of the capacity to satisfy
basic needs and desires. For me as well as Bhaskar, the trio of professional,
policy and critical sociologies does not exhaust its contribution. In fact, on
its own, it diminishes and 'tames' it. Sociology *must* embrace the second trio
of public, foresight and action sociologies.

Transformatory dialectics

To reiterate, 'our ordinary understanding of change involves the *absenting*
of something that was there and/or the *presencing* of something that was not
there. This presencing can also be understood as 'absenting the absence' of
what was not there' (Bhaskar, 2016: 115). This understanding of change incorporates the two key concepts of absence and negativity. Bhaskar (2016: 121)
promotes what he calls an *axiology of freedom*:

> dialectical critical realism seeks to give a real definition of dialectic as
> involving the absenting of absences (including constraints and ills); and
> more especially as absenting absences (qua constraints) on absenting
> absences ((qua ills (which may also be regarded as constraints)) – or, in
> effect, the 'axiology of freedom'.

Bhaskar is also at pains to contextualise his ontological absenting analysis
of change so as to incorporate changes in the beliefs we hold. These beliefs
cannot, he says, be extruded from the world but must rather be part of it,
and therefore susceptible to his ontological analysis. Thus:

> critical realism, in so far as it underlabours for science, must underla-
> bour for a science that deals with changing subject matters, and this
> underlabouring will involve a defence and elaboration of the ideas of
> absence and absenting, negativity and negation in reality, and a defence
> of the categories and concepts we need to understand changes and their
> causes, including the concepts of contradiction (which includes an op-
> position between A and not-A) and other concepts traditionally banned
> from use to describe the world.
>
> (Bhaskar, 2016: 119)

Marmot's reports on health inequalities may be understandably, even commendably, pragmatic and 'performative' – that is, oriented to Popperian
'piecemeal social engineering' and what he would promote as 'realistic', positive shifts in national and global governance – but we have seen that they are
characterised too by the absences of: (a) the *real* (in Bhaskar's sense) mechanisms that deliver health inequalities and (b) any reference to (a). These absences are consonant with and helpful to financial capitalism's class-based and
command-operationalised rentier interests and the neoliberal ideology that

rationalises them. (I want to add here that I do not for a moment underestimate Marmot's committed and noble efforts over decades to inspire change).

A little more needs to be said of Bhaskar's dialectic of freedom, which extends his early tranformational model of social action. We are, he avers, simultaneously acting creatures and judging and speaking beings; 'but our agency has discursive presuppositions and our judgements practical ones' (Bhaskar, 2016: 134–135):

> dialectical critical realism's 'dialectic of freedom' (or 'dialectic of desire to freedom') argues that we can derive the formal criteria for the good society, involving the free flourishing of each as a condition for the free flourishing of all, from either our agency or our discourse alone. We can do this by means of either (1) a 'dialectic of agency' (or of desire and agency) or (2) a 'dialectic of discourse' (or of judgement and speech action or discourse). Substantively, this involves a 'totalising depth-praxis', including research, tending in the direction of universal free flourishing and implied by the research. The combination of formal and substantive criteria, and the dialectical cross-fertilisation of each, issues in 'dialectical reason', or the 'coherence of theory and practice in practice'.

Bhaskar (2016: 135) proceeds to encapsulate this as follows: 'absence – elemental desire – referential detachment – constraint – understanding of the causes of constraint – dialectic of solidarity (immanent critique and dialectical universalisability) – totalising depth praxis – emancipatory axiology.'

The dialectic of desire/agency trades on the conceptual and quasi-propositional nature of desire and intentional agency, plus the fact that desire – want, need – entails a 'meta-desire' for the removal of constraints on its satisfaction. This takes us into the domain of discourse and sociality/solidarity, specifically the desires, wants, needs of others. For all his silence on ontology, there is more than a hint of Habermas here (see Chapter 2). In desiring something, Bhaskar argues, we are committed to

> the removal of constraints, including power 2 or master-slave-type relations, on the satisfaction of the desire, and thus to the removal of all dialectically similar constraints … If I exclude any human being from my concern to remove constraints, I define myself by that relation of exclusion and so limit my own freedom. Freedom is dialectically indivisible
> (Bhaskar, 2016: 135)

The dialectic of speech/discourse, in contrast, trades on the evaluative and practical implications of factual discourse and its trustworthiness ('trust me, you can act on it'). This returns us to sociality/solidarity, 'for to say "trust me, you can act on it" is to say that in your circumstances we ourselves would do it, and this commits us to acting in solidarity with all such addressees' (Bhaskar, 2016: 136).

What implications does this have for the sociology of health inequalities? The title of Bhaskar's posthumous volume is a clue: *Enlightened Common Sense*. The most successful scientists, he contends, have been critical realists without knowing it. The *prediction* and public health-oriented, neo-positivistic social epidemiological research programme of Marmot and colleagues – despite too often, I have maintained, co-opting and 'taming' companionable or funding-dependent medical sociologists – might with profit reflect on this and build on the underlabouring philosophy of basic and dialectical critical realism. I doubt they would contest the retroductive inference to generative mechanisms in the interests of *explaining* health inequalities, whether on the part of the natural, life or social sciences (though they would surely, if erroneously, baulk at the role of abductive inference). Nor would Marmot and other 'scientists' demur from Bhaskar's aspirations for a 'good society' characterised by an equitable distribution of life-chances, health and wellbeing, for all that they might hesitate to sign up to DCR to give voice to them.

What has been on (slow boiling) offer throughout this volume is a neo-Marxist theory of power 2 relations pertinent for explaining the obdurate maldistrubution of health and longevity. Power 2 relations organise, rationalise and enforce 'an "uneven" distribution of the capacity of human agents to exercise transformative power over their conditions of existence and subtract from their autonomy' (Scambler & Scambler, 2015: 348). They negate most people's desires, wants and needs. Bhaskar's dialectic of freedom can be seen as a process of acting to absent constraining ills, and to act to absent constraining ills is to presuppose universal human emancipation. If this thesis can bear their weight, and I think it can, there are numerous sequelae. It is plainly not just that notions like absence and negation possess the critical potential to expose generative mechanisms unintentionally or, more likely with respect to power 2 relations, *intentionally* missing, hidden from view or buried purposefully deep. Nor is it even that they can inspire and afford the means to open up and critique those political and cultural discourses and recipes for action that service neoliberal ideology and function as conduits – and win time and space – for financial capitalism's class/command dynamic. In other words, DCR's promise extends beyond refreshing, contextualising and deepening Marmot-like accounts. DCR provides an ontology and a frame for a credible and appropriately stratified research programme on health inequalities, as well as for a more limited *sociology of health inequalities*. It also underpins and supports the potential of power 1 relations to address, confront and 'transform' that constellation of *really existing* mechanisms that professional, policy and critical sociologies as well as social epidemiology have bypassed (in short, to absent constraining ills deriving from power 2 relations).

Public, foresight and action sociologies remain underdeveloped but could grow to facilitate the sociological project of lifeworld rationalisation (see Table 2.2 in Chapter 2). Public sociology alone is limited. It is in fact reasonable to postulate a *law of inverse salience for social transformation*:

the greater the salience of sociology's contributions for social transformation, the higher the chance that they will be ignored, sidelined, kicked into the long grass or, if push comes to shove, rubbished by tabloid proprietors and editors. Foresight and, in particular, action sociology offer more counterfactual thrust. Consider foresight sociology for example, a form of intervention especially reliant on the use of the sociological imagination. Under this rubric, sociologists might open up and respond to a plethora of 'what if' conjectures and scenarios consequent on ideas of absence and absenting of constraining ills. What would happen if genuine attempts were made to tackle health inequalities via the systematic removal of capital from the exploitative networks of the capital executive and power from the oppressive networks of the political elite from whom they buy policy and on whom they rely for its implementation and enforcement? How, indeed, might such attempts be even launched? How might a crisis of legitimation serious enough to impact on our resilient and well-armed system of parliamentary capitalism be promoted? And on what prospectus? How might a society 'beyond neoliberal ideology' be conceived, rendered concrete and articulated in terms of an extra-parliamentary narrative capable of gaining popular assent? More specifically, what are the alternate, optimum institutional means for delivering not only greater wealth and income equality but better public health and health and social care?

Action sociology is more readily associated with Habermas's (1984, 1987) strategic than with his communicative action, which presages risk as well as opportunity. To contest ideological attacks, it is not enough to simply replicate one's research findings or to disseminate them more widely, although both these are positive (see Wilkinson & Pickett, 2009). The focused autonomous reflexives dominating Britain's governing oligarchy and their establishment allies will not cede ground to reason and evidence alone, having made a speciality of propaganda rooted in policy-based evidence. Nor is it a cliché, as Brexit and the election of Trump in the USA testify, and as we shall see in the final chapters, to suggest that we now inhabit a 'post-truth society'. To enter combat armed only with communicative reason is to do so with one hand tied behind one's back. So, it seems that it is either public 'leading to' foresight and action sociology, or it is a settling for professional, policy and critical sociology and a likely widening of the gap between the health and life expectancy of those – vulnerable fractured reflexives – characterised by a clustering of weak asset flows for health and the exploiters and oppressors to whom they owe their lot.

Considerable portions of this chapter and of those preceding it have been devoted to precis of Bhaskar's basic and dialectical critical realism and to Archer on morphogenesis and reflexivity. I have argued throughout that this formal or philosophical/theoretical input is justified to the extent that it pays off substantively. Given my assertion that the extant sociology of health inequalities is theoretically etiolated and substantively neo-positivistic and inclined to co-option by social epidemiology, it is down to me to show that the investment has been worthwhile and allows us to move on. The final chapters are therefore less philosophical and esoteric. Chapter 6 picks up on the notion of dialectical diagnostics and is an attempt to fashion an overview of Britain – a 'fractured society' – in the era I have named financial capitalism. The point of this overview is to set up and outline a macro- via meso- to micro-sociology of health inequalities that is fit for purpose.

The focus of Chapter 7 is on dialectical transformation. Taking as points of reference rival theories of financial capitalism and social change, it considers structural and cultural obstacles to transformative change as well as alternate routes to its accomplishment. The accent is on the absenting of absence as well as the absenting of constraining ills. It is a perhaps a precursor to or prototypical exercise in foresight and action sociology. It is one thing to capture the principal social mechanisms shaping our lives, another to shape them to our collective, universal benefit. Finally, Chapter 8 sets out a manifesto for a sociology in the twenty-first century.

Part III

6 'Fractured society'

Health and the mechanisms that matter most

We inhabit worlds that are multiply structured and open. Against structured odds we can change things, but rarely do they turn out as we envisage. It is not for nothing that classical versions of sociology often defined it in terms of the unintended consequences of our actions. Moreover, (a) 'we' are each of us an emergent amalgam of the social, psychological and biological; and (b) we are much more likely to reproduce than to transform the multiplicity of structures that define us and into which we were inserted natally. The social scientist's task could scarcely be more dauntingly complex. And yet, as countless sociologists have shown and are showing, there are ways of moving forward. This chapter is an attempt to outline various ways in which the broad brush or macro-characteristics of contemporary societies like Britain play out in peoples' lives, decision-making and health.

What I have throughout referred to as post-1970s financial capitalism has attracted numerous and colourful rival epithets. Some narratives have centred on a putative closure of modernity, others on novel sets of structural, cultural or organisational constellations. It has become commonplace to sum up present day societies, western or otherwise, under rubrics far more audacious than 'financial capitalism'. Capitalism has been described, or proscribed, as predatory or as a global or super 'casino'. Most accounts have incorporated notions of 'acceleration' (though acceleration, qua discourse, now has a life of its own). Archer, it will be remembered, suspects we are on the cusp of a 'morphogenetic society'. Giddens (1990) warned of a juggernaut out of control. Occasionally such overviews have settled and matured somewhat. Critical expositions of a handful of themes or core concepts from such overviews follow. They provide contexts, frames of reference and motivations for my own summary thoughts. I shall make a case that financial capitalism has produced what I shall term a *fractured society*. Many overviews of contemporary society are indebted to the classic schools/theories sketched in Chapter 2, as will become apparent. They are: (a) Zizeck and class struggle, (b) Ritzer and 'McDonaldisation', (c) Bauman and liquid modernity, (d) Castells and network society and (e) Tyler, Scambler and the weaponising of stigma in neoliberalism.

(a) Zizek and class struggle

As we have seen, Marx singled out one prime societal antagonism and referred to it as 'class stuggle'. This, as Zizek discerns, is 'the wager of capitalism'. Class struggle overdetermines all others: it is the 'concrete universal' of the entire field'. Zizek (2016: 60–61) continues:

> the term 'overdetermination' is here used in its precise Althusserian sense. It does not mean that class struggle is the ultimate referent and horizon of meaning of all other struggles. It means that class struggle is the structuring principle that allows us to account for the very 'inconsistent' plurality of ways in which other antagonisms can be articulated into 'chains of equivalences'. For example, feminist struggle can be articulated into a chain with the progressive struggle for emancipation, or it can (and certainly does) function as an ideological tool of the upper-middle classes to assert their superiority over the 'patriarchal and intolerant' lower classes. And the point here is not only that the feminist struggle can be articulated in different ways within the class antagonism, but that class antagonism is as it were doubly inscribed here: it is the specific constellation of the class struggle itself that explains why the feminist struggle was appropriated by the upper-middle classes. (The same goes for racism: it is the dynamics of class struggle itself that explain why direct racism is strong among the lowest white workers.) Class struggle is here the 'concrete universality' in the strict Hegelian sense. In relating to its otherness (other antagonisms), it relates to itself, which is to say that it (over-) determines the way it relates to other struggles.

This quotation from Zizek is a prolegomenon. It introduces several contextualising propositions that require spelling out to avoid misunderstandings. This volume presents a sociology of health inequalities via – it is contended – financial capitalism's most potent generative mechanism for this, as well as many other, social phenomena, namely, the class/command dynamic. Class and command are fundamental to capitalism in all its guises, I have maintained, whereas gender and ethnicity are not. This privileging of class and command (or state) relations is: (a) consonant with the evidence and warranted and (b) in need of qualification. The first point under (b) is a recognition that gender and ethnic or race relations alike *preceeded* the onset of mercantilism/capitalism. Capitalism was as a result gendered and racialised from the outset. Their functionality for capitalism was contingent rather than necessary. It does not follow, and this is the second observation, either that class and command relations can rightfully be said to subsume or annul those of gender and ethnicity, or that the class/command dynamic holds sway *across all contexts or figurations*. Gender and ethnic relations (plus others, including age for example) are causally salient for health inequalities *in their own right*.

To many commentators, sexism and racism appear more potent in financial capitalism than 'classism': class as a social structure or relation no longer translates as easily or smoothly into class-consciousness and clas-sism as it did even a generation ago (during postwar welfare capitalism). In his remarkable *Why We Can't Afford the Rich*, Sayer (2015) highlights the continuing significance of sexism, racism (and disablism) and their contri-butions to '*unfair* inequalities', based primarily on various forms of preju-dice and discrimination. He expands:

> while gender and race inequalities are produced primarily by sexism and racism, class differences would persist even if the upper and middle classes were nice and respectful to the working class. The unequal distribution of property and the unequal division of labour would be largely unaffected. Class prejudice is common, but it's more a 'response to' economic ine-qualities than a cause of them. By contrast, the enduring of sexism and racism would have a major impact on gender and race inequalities.
>
> (Sayer, 2015: 170)

Sayer acknowledges that gender and ethnic inequalities *can* be the product of structural features. Groups can be trapped in poor neighbourhoods less by any prejudice against them than by their inability to afford better hous-ing. Predominant among the 'structural features' that feed into gender and ethnic inequalities, however, are the unequal division of labour and inequal-ities in pay and property ownership.

Competitive forces will take advantage of any inequalities they can, for example in their pursuit of cheap labour. But capitalism does not *need* ine-qualities of gender and ethnicity: 'there are plenty of other ways of making a profit'. What employers need are 'workers' (of whatever gender, ethnic group):

> ... and they do need control over the means of production. Capitalism is not dependent for its very existence on these other sources of inequality, but it does depend on controlling the means of production.
>
> (Sayer, 2015: 170)

Sayer continues:

> this is why equal opportunity policies are usually quite good on gender, race, age, sexuality, religion and disability, but silent on economic class.

'Enlightened' employers don't even pretend to challenge 'structural class differences' (Sayer, 2015: 170). No more, I might add, do most socio-epidemiologically inclined sociologists researching and writing on health inequalities. A final quote from Sayer (2015: 170):

> Neoliberals – New Labour for example – can appear quite progressive about gender, race, sexuality, disability and condemn those who dis-criminate against people on these grounds. Unsurprisingly, the elephant

in the room is economic inequalities or class differences. Though it never admits it, neoliberalism is a political-economic movement that seeks to legitimise widening economic inequalities and defend rentier interests above all others. Rentiers can live off others regardless of their gender, race, sexuality and so on.

• Zizek and Sayer address the issue of putting all the eggs of health inequalities into the one class and command basket. My argument is that the class/command dynamic is *the* prepotent mechanism for a sociology of health inequalities in the figuration of the British nation state. I am *not* suggesting, however, either that it is the prepotent mechanism across all figurations or that it is the sole mechanism in the figuration of the nation state. This would be foolish. I once espoused what I called the 'jigsaw model' (see Scambler, 2002, 2005b). This had three components, the first being a 'best guess' at the *overall picture* of the dynamic, complex and highly differentiated social world we inhabit; the second a series of models articulated in terms of *logics*, *relations* and *figurations* (each constituting a discrete piece of the jigsaw); and the third a process of *dialectical reasoning* by means of which the sense of the overall picture informs the application of models and the application of models informs the sense of the overall picture. Deploying this frame, I am contending here that if we are after a sociological explanation of health inequalities in the figuration of the British nation state, then, borrowing from French regulation theory, the key logics are Habermas's subsystems of the economy (the regime of capital accumulation) and the state (mode of regulation). These logics give rise to relations of class and command, respectively. Hence, the focus in this contribution on the class/command dynamic. This is, as it were, a particularly important piece of a large and tricky multi-piece jigsaw. But there are of course multiple other figurations – regional, local, communities, estates, neighbourhoods, households and so on – and in these the 'key' logics and relations can, and do, differ. In some, for example, it is the logic of patriarchy and relations of gender that are paramount.

(b) Ritzer and 'McDonaldization'

Capitalism necessarily entails an open urge and aspiration to commodification until there is nothing beyond the grasp of its tentacles. If the air we breathe could be afforded an exchange value, why not? What I have called financial capitalism has often been referred to as 'consumer society'. Ritzer's contribution was to link this ever-expanding commodification, currently being foisted onto the NHS as we have seen, to the process exemplified in fast-food preparation and delivery. Thus, McDonaldisation refers to 'the process by which the principles of the fast-food restaurant are coming to dominate more and more sectors of American society, as well as the rest of the world' (Ritzer, 2003: 138). Ritzer identified five basic dimensions: *efficiency, calculability, predictability, control through the substitution of technology for people* and, paradoxically, *the irrationality of rationality*.

A McDonaldising society emphasises efficiency, the kind of instrumentalism that always opts for the optimum means to a chosen end. Workers in fast-food outlets work in assembly-line fashion, and customers are likewise expected to consume efficiently. The drive-through window is the epitome of this form of consumption. In Ritzer's (2003: 139) words:

> overall, a variety of norms, rules, regulations, procedures, and structures have been put in place in the fast-food restaurant in order to ensure that 'both' employees and customers act in an efficient manner. Furthermore, the efficiency of one party helps to ensure that the other will behave in a similar manner.

Calculability privileges quantity over quality. It often leads to employee dissatisfaction, alienation and a high staff turnover. Customers too are hurried and harried. McDonalds cannot, and do not, provide a high-quality dining experience. With calculability comes predictability. Employees and customers are required to follow their scripts and behave as expected, and somewhat ritualistically. This, in turn, marries with control. A McDonalised environment is characterised by modes of control that issue from technologies. While employees are controlled by such technologies as 'french-fry machines', customers are constrained by their own and employees' scripts and routines and by the automated technologies too: just try ordering, Ritzer remarks, 'well-done, well-browned fries'. Moreover, technology threatens to replace humans in a plethora of McDonalised workplaces.

Finally, both employees and customers, Ritzer contends, are afflicted by the irrationality of rationality. What does he mean by this? He points out a number of minor irrationalities, like the inefficient queueing that compromises what is intended, presented and celebrated as a paradigmatically efficient service. But he has in mind something deeper: 'the ultimate irrationality of rationality is dehumanization' (Ritzer, 2003: 141). Workers and customers are compelled to work in dehumanizing jobs and to eat in dehumanizing settings, respectively. 'The fast-food restaurant is a source of degradation for employees and customers alike' (Ritzer, 2003: 141).

McDonalds, as the model of the process of McDonaldisation, has come to occupy a pivotal position worldwide. It has become a global phenomenon. Hence:

> the McDonalidization thesis is that McDonald's and, more importantly, the principles that lie at its bases ... are affecting increasingly more sectors of society and more parts of the world. The image is of a society and a world in which it is increasingly hard to find non-McDonaldized settings. This image is an updated version of Weber's thesis that the world was

moving inexorably in the direction of an iron cage of rationalization. We are far closer to that iron cage than we were in Weber's day and the process is better caught by the term 'McDonaldization' than 'rationalization'.

(Ritzer, 2003: 144)

• What to take from Ritzer's thesis? Whilst accepting Habermas's argument that Weber's insistence on the 'inexorability' of an emergent iron cage of rationalization was misplaced (lifeworld rationalization was and remains a realizable alternative), it is clear that the McDonalisation process, a form of systemic colonization of the lifeworld, has *in fact* proceeded apace. Check out US health care. And it is a process that is currently being translated not only into multiple British workplaces but is allied to the alpha-male, white, 'greedy bastardised' privatisation of the NHS. The likes of Branson offer a McDonaldised, profitable 'solution' to NHS conundrums strategically delivered by our governing oligarchy. This is financial capitalism's revised version of Fordism. Emphasising the impact and reach of contemporary transnational corporations, Monbiot (2016) maintains that 'no country with a McDonalds can remain a democracy'. Interest here too is in what might lie ahead, notably with the introduction of robots into the McDonaldised process.

(c) Bauman and liquid modernity

Bauman's intellectual trajectory is complex and intriguing. I bypass here his earlier work, including his superb, prize-winning *Modernity and the Holocaust*, to focus on the manner of his accommodation to theories of postmodernism and postmodernity. Ritzer (2003: 243) presciently notes that 'he can be thought of as *either* a modern *or* a postmodern social theorist'. Bauman generally favours a sociology of the postmodern/postmodernity over a postmodern sociology (though this is not always clear). He stresses the contemporary challenge to adapt to 'ambivalence'. Our postmodern culture, he suggests, opens up new possibilities and new dangers in this respect. On a positive note, there is a postmodern acceptance of the messiness of the world. Yet, this heralds a new level of multiple uncertainties. Moreover, these uncertainties have become individualised or 'private' matters:

faced with private fears, postmodern individuals are also doomed to try to escape those fears on their own. Not surprisingly, they have been drawn to communities as shelters from these fears. However, this raises the possibility of conflict between communities. Bauman worries about these hostilities and argues that we need to put a brake on them through the development of solidarity.

(Ritzer, 2003: 243)

In an era characterised as 'neotribal', I would add that it is unsurprising that people who find themselves 'deserted' and 'alone' in a postmodern, relativised culture seek refuge in fundamentalisms, an issue to which we shall return (what kind of toleration is it that tolerates fundamentalisms?).

Ritzer (2003: 246) reports that Bauman outlines four principal forms of contemporary politics. The first is 'tribal politics', which asserts that postmodern tribes exist symbolically as imagined communities; and these tribes compete via rituals and spectacles to win approval and support. The second is a 'politics of desire', which refers to tribes' commitment to and commendation of certain types of behaviour. It is a politics of seduction: tribes compete to lodge their tokens in people's minds as objects of desire. Third is the 'politics of fear', which derives from a scepticism and mistrust of the pronouncements and counsel of assorted political agencies. Finally comes the 'politics of certainty', which encompasses a mistrust of those 'experts' who, if only they could (still) be trusted, might proffer solutions to pressing problems of purpose and self-identity.

Many of these ideas and claims are epitomised in Bauman's (2000) concept of 'liquid modernity'. Revealingly, the subtitle of his *Liquid Times* is 'living in an age of uncertainty (Bauman, 2007). I concentrate here on his remarks on freedom. A distinction is made between subjective and objective freedom. Subjective freedom has to do with how one perceives the limits to one's freedom, while objective freedom pertains, when all's said and done, to one's *actual* capacity to act. Thus, people can feel (subjectively) either free or constrained in contradiction with their (objective) circumstances. Bauman suggests that people can and do dislike the idea of freedom because it seems a 'mixed blessing'. He is not unsympathetic, citing Durkheim's judgement that by putting oneself under the wings of society one might gain a 'liberating dependence'. To be totally free is to exist in a constant agony of uncertainty and indecision, not least in relation to the will of others. Norms provide welltrod paths and settled routines. Contemporary societies remain open to critique, but the context and targets have changed. Critiques have shifted from positing and promoting societal change to a focus on ourselves and our lifepolitics. Our reflexivity has become shallow and no longer extends meaningfully to the systemness of society or the system's colonisation of the lifeworld.

In liquid modernity the options to disavow one's individualism and to decline to participate have been removed. How one lives adds up to a biographical solution to systemic contradictions. The contradictions and their associated risks remain, but the duty to confront and deal with them has become individualised and a matter of personal responsibility. Bauman (2000) argues too that a gap is opening up between individuality as fate and the capacity for self-assertion. This 'capacity', he suggests, now falls well short of what is required for genuine, 'authentic' self-assertion. It is the task of a 'critical theory of society', Bauman avers, to devise the means to so empower individuals that they have a degree of control over the resources required for authentic self-assertion.

• Bauman is such a prolific writer that the preceding paragraphs cannot be said to afford a precis of his (evolving) thesis; but they are a purposeful extraction. What is important is that: (a) when push comes to shove, he opts for a commitment to continuity as opposed to discontinuity by retaining the concept of 'modernity'; and (b) he catches much of the cultural change that has accompanied, and is functional for, financial capitalism. Both (a) and (b) warrant elaboration. It will be apparent from Chapter 2 that I am unconvinced by arguments for the end of modernity (let alone of history). I have avoided the prejudicial term 'late modernity' and used the more neutral 'high modernity' (Scambler & Higgs, 1999). Bauman also distanced himself (eventually) from conjectures around a new era of postmodernity. Capitalism persists, if in innovative clothing, as do so many of its social structures/relations/mechanisms. However, Bauman perspicuously analyses the cultural transumutation that has walked in tandem with financial capitalism. This novel ('rejoice, you're on your own') postmodern relativism, which Habermas wisely casts as the latest form of neo-conservatism, delivers significant obstacles to the solidarity that Bauman calls for. *The* key question for sociology in my view is this: how in this most unsympathetic and inauspicious phase of financial capitalism can the objective reality of class relations and struggle or 'warfare' be translated into a potentially belligerent and transformative subjective sense of, and impulse to, 'class consciousness'? Bauman's contribution is to lay bare the cultural 'obstacles' (see also Bauman, 2011).

(d) Castells and network society

Castells is another eminent theorist of society and social change whose work is relevant here. The foci of much of his work are information and communication power in the context of network society. He insists on preserving the analytical distance and empirical relation between modes of production (capitalism, statism) and modes of development (industrial, informational) (Castells, 1996). The source of productivity in the present informational mode of development lies in the technology of knowledge generation, information processing and symbolic communication. What I call financial capitalism he calls 'informational capitalism'; and he defines it as a novel 'techno-economic system' characterised by flexibility and adaptability. This, then, is a new mode of production that heralds an expansion and rejuvenation of capitalism. Williams (2012: 171) expands:

> within this new economy moreover, a premium is placed on flexible, adaptable 'self-programmable' flows of labour able to 'autonomously process information into specific knowledge' vis-à-vis 'generic workers'

who must be 'ready to adapt to the needs of this new economy or else face displacement by machines or alternative labour forces'.

(Castells, 2009: 33)

Wisely, Castells admits to considerable heterogeneity in societal accommodations of 'informationalism'.

He goes on to differentiate two ways actors can influence their consociates: (a) by means of *coercion* (or the threat of it); and (b) by means of the *construction of meaning*, that is, the shaping of those discourses that inform actors' actions. Power, he asserts:

> relies on the control of communication, as counter power depends on the breaking of such control. And mass communication, the communication that potentially reaches society at large, is shaped and managed by power relationships, rooted in the business of media and the politics of the state.
>
> (Castells, 2009: 3)

It is an analysis that resonates not only with Bhaskar's power 2 relations, but with Habermas's notion of the system's continuing colonisation, or 'refeudalisation', of the public sphere of the lifeworld. Castells comments on new social movements in this context. He relates these to two of three ideal types of identity. The first 'unrelated' type is 'legitimising identity', which is engineered by dominant interests (such as the class/command dynamic) and by and large reproduces the status quo. The second type is 'resistance identity', 'generated by those actors who are in positions/ conditions devalued and/or stigmatised by the logic of domination, thus building trenches of resistance and survival on the basis of principles different from, or opposed to, those permeating the institutions of society' (Castells, 2010a,b: 8). The accent here is on the 'exclusion of the excluders by the excluded' (see Williams, 2012: 173). The third type is 'project identity', denoting a situation in which social actors 'build a new identity that redefines their position in society and, by doing so, seek the transformation of overall social structure' (Castells, 2010a,b: 8). The end sought is integration through the transformation of extant ruling institutions, norms and values (e.g. the feminist opposition to patriarchal 'logic').

The state under financial capitalism has also undergone significant change, culminating in a 'network state'. Flexible governance is key, while the political domain is characterised by 'informational politics'. Political parties lost salience in the face of the (new) media system. The media system, and especially the electronic media, filter all political decision-making. Hence communicative power is the fundamental form of power in the information age. The exercise of this power results in *exclusion* rather than domination or repression. Flows of information simply bypass and render marginal and redundant large segments of the world's populations. Thus 'black holes' are commonplace, ranging from the ghettoes hidden behind American cities to what Castells calls the 'fourth world' of the African continent (Williams, 2012).

Networks have always existed, but not as the dominant form of social organization, and never in their present 'technologically facilitated, information driven, form' (Williams, 2012: 174). A 'network logic' now permeates lives in all their complexity. Informationalism and networking are 'intimately yet *contingently* connected in *complex, dynamic, reciprocal, mutually reinforcing* ... ways – informationalism being a technological matter, networking a question of social morphology ...' (Williams, 2012: 175). Moreover, time and space have been transformed, encouraging Castells to write of the 'space of flows'. The space of flows refers to the material organization of time-sharing practices that function through flows. This alludes to the rapidly expanding role of new electronic circuits and continuous flows of communication – '*at a distance* yet in *simultaneous time* – in the information age and the network society' (Williams, 2012: 175).

The notion of a space of flows is further broken down into three aspects. The first is a 'circuit of electronic exchanges' (comprising micro-electronics-based, telecommunications, computer processing, broadcasting systems etc); the second is the 'nodes and hubs' that make up information networks; and the third is the spatial organization of the dominant managerial elites – *not* classes – that 'exercise the directional functions around which such space is articulated' (Williams, 2012: 175). The space of flows, Castells notes, does not penetrate the lifeworld as a whole. This leads him to refer also to a 'space of places'. Most people most of the time (still) experience their space as place-based. The spaces of flows and places remain in tension. Yet:

> ... because function and power in our societies are organized in the space of flows, the structural domination of its logic essentially alters the meaning and dynamics of places. Experience, by being related to spaces, becomes abstracted from power and meaning is increasingly separated from knowledge. There follows a structural schizophrenia logic that threatens to break down communication channels in society. The dominant tendency is toward a horizon of networked, ahistorical space of flows, aiming at imposing its logic over scattered, segmented places, increasingly unrelated to each other, less and less able to share cultural codes
>
> (Castells, 2000: 458–459)

Williams (2012: 179) addresses Castells's neglect of national and transnational concepts of class. Forgive me if I cite him at some length since his statement on Castells reasoning is particularly lucid:

> to think or speak in such terms ... for Castells, would be to mistakenly attribute agency and control to a 'class' or group who themselves

are caught up, and hence subject to, the 'mighty whirlwind' of faceless capitalism and the uncertainties of global financial markets: a complex, constantly changing configuration or reconfiguration of power and networks, that is to say. Conflict moreover is no longer primarily articulated around questions and issues to do with who owns the means of production. Castells then in this regard, as Stalder (2006: 191) comments, appears more comfortable speaking of a 'global elite' than a capitalist or global class, with a focus on a 'shared culture' facilitated through communication in the global networks of power and wealth.

For all the richness and topicality of Castells's studies, it will have been apparent from my earlier comments on elite analysis that I reject the growing, neo-Foucauldian tendency in twenty-first-century sociological circles to pass on class. I shall return to Castells, but to avoid confusion will here reiterate my view that: (a) it has become too easy to neglect structural continuities in the face of the onslaughts of financial capitalism's putatively accelerating cultural discontinuities; (b) considered objectively, class is more germane and potent in financial than it was in postwar welfare capitalism; (c) considered subjectively, the input of class into identity-formation, and therefore its possible transmutation into an energised and oppositional form of class consciousness, has diminished since the mid-1970s; and (d) the conflation of class structures or relations with culture, epitomised in the Great British Class Survey and the notion of a new 'class paradigm', is as misguided for sociologists and those languishing in relative poverty as it is an effective camouflage for the beneficiaries of the class/command dynamic.

(e) Tyler, Scambler and the weaponising of stigma in neoliberalism

In his popular bestseller *Chavs*, Owen Jones (2011) put together a telling account – its roots somehow lost in Goffman's (1968b) time-honoured dramaturgical explication of stigma – of how financial capitalism has witnessed the shaming or 'othering' of a whole segment of the British population. As Tyler (2013) has vividly shown, this extends beyond the preaching of billionaire, tax-evading, proprietor-sponsored tabloid indignation to feature in mainstream media mockery: witness the routine TV stereotyping of a supposedly benefit-sapping underclass in so-called reality shows. What has emerged is the political exclusion or casting out – Tyler (2013) uses the term 'social abjection' – of collectivities of the undeserving and vulnerable. These include Jones's 'chavs', but Tyler writes also of asylum seekers, gypsies and travellers. She links their marginalisation with the financial capitalism's neoliberal ideology. If collectivities can be successfully reconstructed as abject, after all, they can be ignored, sidelined, sanctioned and even punished. During Cameron's Tory regime in Britain, 2010–2015, Ian Duncan Smith came most to symbolise this calculated policy of redefining those most harmed by the no less calculated policy of austerity, namely, the poor, unemployed, benefit 'seekers' (or 'shirkers'), plus the long-term sick or disabled, as abject and – after Foucault – personally responsible and liable for any hardship (Scambler, In Press).

Tyler (Forthcoming) has since switched her attention to consolidating and expanding the sociology of stigma post-Goffman. Klein (2007) has written of the ways in which what she calls the paramount 'policy trinity' of (a) neoliberalism, (b) the calculated decimation of the public sphere and (c) the total liberation for corporations and skeletal welfare spending, has been oiled by the invention and/or exploitation of crises or shocks, for example natural disasters and terrorist attacks. Tyler's own focus is currently on 'the ways in which neoliberal modes of government operate not only by capitalizing upon 'shocks' but through the daily, pervasive production and mediation of stigma'. Stigma, it might be said, is being *weaponised* for political ends.

My own recent studies of stigma are in a similar vein. They build on an earlier distinction between stigma and deviance (Scambler, 2009; Scambler, Forthcoming). Stigma, I have maintained, might usefully be regarded as an offence against norms of *shame*, while deviance might be seen as an offence against norms of *blame*. Table 6.1 presents a breakdown of my concepts of enacted, felt and project stigma and deviance. Enacted stigma and deviance denote actual discrimination due to failures of conformance and compliance respectively. Felt stigma and deviance refer to internalisations of shame and blame and the fear, inhibiting in its own right, of encountering enacted stigma and deviance. Finally, project stigma and deviance allow for the often-neglected potential for people to resist enacted and felt stigma and deviance (Table 6.1).

To these distinctions, I have appended a quartet of ideal types reflecting extant sociocultural norms of shame and blame. These overlap with, yet can be distinguished from, Tyler's ongoing project. The logic is simple. Four classes

Table 6.1 Notions of Stigma and Deviance

STIGMA *(offences against norms of shame)*	**DEVIANCE** *(offences against norms of blame)*
Enacted stigma	*Enacted deviance*
Actual discrimination (shaming)	Actual discrimination (blaming)
Felt stigma	*Felt deviance*
Fear of discrimination and sense of shame	Fear of discrimination and sense of blame
Project stigma	*Project deviance*
Active resistance to enacted and felt stigma	Active resistance to enacted and felt deviance

Table 6.2 Stigma and/or Deviance, Shame and/or Blame

Stigma + Deviance + *Abjects*	Stigma + deviance − *Rejects*
Stigma − deviance − *Normals*	Stigma − Deviance + *Losers*

are framed as follows: (1) stigma + deviance +, (2) stigma + deviance −, (3) stigma − deviance − and (4) stigma − deviance +. For convenience and bite, I label these, respectively, *abjects*, *rejects*, *normals* and *losers*. They are reproduced in Table 6.2.

Three of these classes/labels, each constructing, announcing and 'performing' abnormality, are as grim as it is to be consigned to any of them. Nobody aspires to be dismissed or 'policed' as an abject, reject or loser. What Tyler's and my accounts have in common is the notion that stigma has become weaponised in neoliberalism (Scambler, In Press). In my own terminology, charges of deviance (blame) have been appended to charges of stigma (shame) and calculatingly deployed to rationalise/legitimise action against the disadvantaged and vulnerable. Tyler stresses, however, phenomena that I have hitherto neglected, namely, project stigma and deviance: it is possible to resist and to fight back.

Fractured society

I have spelled out why and how I judge the class/command dynamic to be *the* mechanism for financial capitalism; and I have indicated why and how it is no less pivotal for a sociology of health inequalities. But the identification and characterisation of the post-1970s capitalist 'phase' does not exhaust the sociology of a much-changed and changing society. The contours of financial capitalism are not the same as those of what I here call our fractured society. Just as, for Castells, the space of flows does not so invade the territory of the lifeworld as to entirely eliminate the space of places, so, to recall Habermas once more, the subsystem of the economy does not so colonise the lifeworld as to render it supine.

But why 'fractured' society? All contemporary societies have hairline cracks, visible or otherwise, in their structures, institutions and organizations, cultures, modes of interaction or across all of these. This is part of the complex messiness of living in highly differentiated societies and, incidentally, of sociology's partial and limited explanatory capability. Some hairline cracks can open somewhat without posing undue threats to social equilibria. But others, analogous to fissures in the weight-bearing walls of a house, require monitoring and speedy remedial action in the event of threats of fracture. This is a roundabout way of saying that Britain – and kindred western societies – are fracturing in ways hazardous to the status quo. The goal in this chapter is circumscribed. It is to offer a sketch of the contours of our fractured society that: (a) extends beyond the analysis of financial capitalism and (b) draws on the theoretical flotsam and jetsam of previous chapters, from the introduction of diverse schools of sociological thinking in Chapter 2 to the elaborations offered thereafter that range from fleeting references to meso- or middle-range theories to sketches of overarching or macro-accounts. Theories about 'crises' and 'post-capitalism' will be addressed in the next chapter.

(a) System disintegration

In a fractured society, there exist cracks within both economic and political (sub)systems. Streeck (2016) draws on Lockwood's (1964) classic distinction between system and social integration, that is, integration at the macro and micro level respectively. Contemporary capitalism, he writes:

> would appear to be a society whose system integration is critically and irremediably weakened, so that the continuation of capital accumulation – for an indeterminate period of uncertain duration – becomes solely dependent on the opportunism of collectively incapacitated 'individualized individuals', as they struggle to protect themselves from looming accidents and structural pressures on their social and economic status. Undergoverned and undermanaged, the social world of the post-capitalist interregnum, in the wake of neoliberal capitalism having cleared away states, governments, borders, trade unions and other moderating forces, can at any time be hit by disaster; for examples bubbles imploding or violence penetrating from a collapsing periphery into the centre. With individuals deprived of collective defences and left to their own devices, what remains of a social order hinges on the motivation of individuals to cooperate with other individuals on an ad hoc basis, driven by fear and greed and by elementary interests in individual survival. Society having lost the ability to provide its members with effective protection and proven templates for social action and social existence, individuals only have themselves to rely on while social order depends on the weakest possible mode of social integration, 'Zweckrationalitat'.
>
> (Streeck, 2016: 14)

Note the reference here to a 'post-capitalist interregnum', reflecting Streeck's thesis that although the future remains uncertain, systemic fissures have opened up beyond repair. A crisis of state legitimation, it seems, is overdue. As we shall return to in detail in the next chapter however, the contradictions of capitalism implicit in Adam Smith and explicit in Marx are, paradoxically, *more salient objectively*, but *less salient subjectively*, in fractured society.

Streeck suggests that this systemic crisis has been germinating for a while. He identifies three trends dating back to the 1970s: declining growth, growing inequality and rising debt (public, private and overall).

Those state-engineered interventions or 'correctives' available to restore the economic status quo during liberal and postwar capitalism now have inadequate purchase. Financial capitalism has so deregulated its regime of capital accumulation as to jeopardise its mode of regulation. So while its class/command dynamic appears in rude and profitable health, there is an underlying system fragility. In Luhmann's terms, the economic system has nudged changes in the political system. Streeck (2016: 58) takes this further: 'the image I have of capitalism – an end that I believe is already underway – is one of a social system in chronic disrepair, for reasons of its own and regardless of the absence of a viable alternative.' He continues:

> social integration as well as system integration seems irreversibly damaged and set to deteriorate further. What is most likely to happen as time passes is a continuous accumulation of small and not-so-small dysfunctions, none necessarily deadly as such, but most beyond repair, all the more so as they become too many for individual address.
>
> (Streeck, 2016: 58)

The fact that there are no apparent successor narratives to capitalism Streeck sees as an additional nail in its coffin, since it has always fed off oppositional conflict.

(b) Class: an absent presence

The transnational capital monopolists, auxiliaries and sleepers that comprise the capitalist executive, together with their new and old middle-class and working-class allies and co-optees, continue to prosper even as precarity seeps its way up from the working class through the old and new middle classes and swathes of the former are 'left behind' (see Table 3.1). These are the beneficiaries of the class/command dynamic. And what benefits at the very top! Even as I write this, Oxfam has announced that eight men now possess as much wealth as the bottom 50% of the global population, that is, 3.6 billion people (one in 10 people worldwide survive on less than $2 per day). Britain's fractured society is riven by class above all else. The extent to which relations of gender and ethnicity promote, consolidate or mitigate class divisions is a figuration-specific and empirical matter; nor is it a simple issue of doubling or tripling 'jeopardy'. However, what the research does indicate is that women and non-white British citizens, migrants or refugees are typically the first to feel the impact of any class tightening of screws. Moreover, the unpredicted phenomenon of the Brexit referendum vote in 2016 unleashed new waves of bitterness and antipathy towards ethnic communities in general and migrants (within which category refugees from Syria and elsewhere were conveniently subsumed) in particular, a social shift 'individualised' as 'hate crime'.

But class, Zizek and Sayers imply, is the elephant in the room. It bites often and deep into the flesh of the citizenry. Yet even as it does so, and for a multiplicity of reasons, it somehow avoids being conspicuous: even sociologists lose sight of it (witness researchers of health inequalities who typically opt for convenient but weak, safe and escapist proxies like socioeconomic group or status), let alone the population as a whole. Even as polls confirm that an increasing majority of British people believe they live in a 'class society', the salience of class for their perceptions of self and self-worth, for identity-formation, for self-for-others and for their day-to-day decision-making and action remains minimal. Class and class struggle, in short, no longer automatically forge class consciousness. As a result, class structure is a dormant, latent force. It is, I shall argue in the next chapter, a fuse waiting to be lit. It constitutes an absent presence, an (objectively) latent mechanism, a tendency, with the potential to become (subjectively) manifest, to be triggered, in the fractured society.

(c) McDonaldised 'end-stage' control

Ritzer presents 'McDonaldisation' as an extension of Habermas's system rationalisation of the lifeworld, an iron cage beyond Weber's imagining. It is reasonable, however, to envision its immediate future as tied to that of financial capitalism itself. If, as Streeck argues, the latter is in an end-stage, then it might be anticipated that the era's standardised mode of control – one exercised through a McDonaldised producer-consumer relationship – will become another fissure set to enlarge. Such a projection, though audacious, is viable even in the face of the current evidence and celebration of transnational processes of McDonaldisation. There is resistance to be sure to the colonising protocols and business models of the likes of McDonalds, Starbucks and so on, but so far with minimal impact. Meanwhile, it is clear that labour costs are ready to be further cut courtesy of advances in artificial intelligence and the infusion of the robot into, and the digitalisation of, producer-consumer relations. It has been estimated that almost 50% of present American jobs could be done by robots, many of them in a burgeoning service sector employing educated high school and university graduates. Financial capitalism's stand-out organizational form, McDonaldisation, is being rolled out and extended even as the system that gave rise to it is imploding.

McDonaldisation is becoming digitalised. It is not in vain that sociologists are prone to refer to 'digital society' or have formed networks to pioneer 'digital sociology' (Lupton, 2016). This represents an astonishingly recent cultural shift:

- World Wide Web: invented 1989, public 1994
- Wikipedia & iTunes, 2001
- LinkedIn, 2003
- Facebook, 2004
- Reddit, Flickr and YouTube, 2005

- Twitter, 2006
- Smartphones, Tumblr, 2007
- Spotify, 2008
- Instagram and Tablet, 2010
- Pinterest and Google+, 2011

But it is also a profound shift, heralding an institutionalisation of flexible routines that might perhaps be characterised in terms of Castells's concept of flows. What is frequently overlooked in all the excitement however is that these are for the most part system generated, friendly and rewarding. While electronic media flows do indeed afford novel opportunities not only for self-presentation and self-marketing but for lifeworld rationalisation in general, and movement activity oriented to lifeworld decolonisation in particular, their primary allegiance is to system needs. They are dutifully responsive to relations of class. Moreover, they are currently being reigned in, undermined by colonising rhetorics of 'post-truth' and 'fake news' and put under surveillance using anti-terrorist legislation passed in the name of national security; command relations in the last resort serve those of class.

In the domain of health, advances in the modes and manner of electronic information flows have Mertonian 'latent' as well as 'manifest functions'. The manifest functions associated with health aps and around what Lupton (2015) calls the 'quantified self' promise a liberating release from old-style bureaucratic health treatment and care, an NHS for the twenty-first century. 'Self-management' is the siren call. It is a call that disguises a set of latent functions. For self-management, read Foucault's 'personal responsibility'; and personal responsibility, as we have seen, is more often than not a gloss for the state's withdrawal from health care (and welfare) provision and its subservience to the capital executive and capital accumulation. Individualised/personalised risk is an aspect of financial capitalism's neoliberal ideology. A logical next step would be personal responsibility/behavioural conditionality leading, via digital implants, to near total surveillance in the service of capital. Fox (2015) discerns corporate, public health, patient and resistant-citizen agendas in these health care innovations. In our fractured society, it is the (latent) corporate agenda that is likely to prevail, resulting in a net loss for citizen-cum-consumers. Luhmann again: behind our backs, digitalisation and 'big data' are via neoliberal ideology scripting or 'modelling' consumers.

(d) Surplus cultural liquidity

It can appear to some twenty first century consumers that there is a surfeit of cultural liquidity, though much of it is in fact funded by individual and household credit underwritten by a state indebtedness, literally and figuratively, to the capitalist executive. Freedom of choice is an illusion, a sleight of hand, a cruel subtext for those less comfortably positioned in the fractured society. Freedom and choice have resource implications.

Moreover excess, 'kalaedoscopic' cultural liquidity can help induce a sense of impotence and passivity. Too many petit narratives and scripts can cancel each other out. Studies of the relativised multiplicity of cultural scripts and repertoires are part cause and part effect of a fascination on the part of sociologists and others with identity-formation, recognition, belonging and so on. It is not that these are unimportant foci for theory and research, more that they have displaced and in the process relegated long established structural concerns. As with recent culturalist approaches to class relations, epitomised in the Great British Class Survey and its progeny, too many babies have disappeared with the bathwater. I am no economic determinist, but it would be strangely neglectful not to record that the cultural appropriation, or deconstruction, of social structures like class, gender and ethnicity is politically convenient and sits comfortably with the ubiquitous ideology of neoliberalism and the politics of the status quo (Habermas, 1989). Consumers are being sold a pup.

(e) Flows and 'superhubs'

I draw on Habermasian terminology again here. There is an understandable tendency for commentators to emphasise the potential of the internet and digitalisation as conduits for lifeworld debate and rationalisation. They promise, it is sometimes claimed, novel forms of resistance to system rationalisation and colonisation. While there is some truth in this, it would be naïve to underestimate the reach and penetration of the steering media of the economy (i.e. money) in the service of an exploitative class push for capital accumulation, and the state (i.e. power) manifest in an oppressive command push for surveillance and control.

Castells's notions of networks and space of flows are particularly apt. They coalesce in what Navidi (2017), a possessor of insider knowledge, calls 'superhubs'. Looking closely at how the nomadic, transnational capital executives ply their trade at the World Economic Forums in Davos, the meetings of the International Monetary Fund, think-tank gatherings and so on, she articulates how bankers, CEOs of transnational corporations, fund managers, rentiers and politicians not only share information and do deals around new troughs to sink their snouts into but – in line with the class/command dynamic – bequeath poverty, disadvantage, diminished health and premature deaths to swathes of the populations with which they are nominally aligned. She writes:

> I began to realise that in a world where everything can be commodified and automated, and in which human interactions are increasingly digitalised, these select few preside over the most exclusive and powerful asset: a unique network of personal relationships that spans the globe, the cultivation of which cannot be delegated or outsourced.
>
> (Navidi, 2017: xxiii–xv)

Contrary to rumour, it is a network characterised more by Mills's tacit understanding than by conscious conspiracy. Navidi names names and institutions:

> with their 'network power', people such as Jamie Dimon, CEO of JP-Morgan Chase; Larry Fink, Chairman and CEO of Blackrock, the largest asset management company in the world; and billionaire hedge fund honcho George Soros shape history, transform the world we live in, and determine the future of our financial system, economy and society.

She continues:

> Heads of central banks – such as the US Federal Reserve, the European Central Bank and the Bank of England – directly impact the interest yield of our savings, the price of out mortgages, and the performance of our pension plans ... Every action of any one of these financiers directly affects the lives of each and every one of us. Through their interconnections with the corporate sector, they increase the individual power exponentially. According to a study by the Swiss Federal Institute of Technology, a select few financial institutions control a large part of the world's biggest companies through cross-holdings and board seats. Because financial institutions consist of individuals, this ownership provides these individuals with enormous influence.

The superhubs comprise a fraction of the 1% of capital monopolists who summon and exercise hugely disproportionate class-based power. Their absence from sociological considerations of health inequalities speaks to a subdiscipline that has been comprehensively 'tamed' (Scambler, 1996). I will argue in the final chapter that this represents a challenge for the whole community of sociologists.

(f) Heaping blame on shame

The (structural) class/command dynamic and its (cultural) sequelae have led to a political 'skewing' of social norms of shame and blame. This is what I term the weaponising of stigma. We have witnessed a historically rapid shift according to which *stigma (norms marking an ontological deficit, non-conformance or shame,) has been redefined as deviance (norms marking a moral deficit, non-compliance or blame)*. Hence the thesis that stigma has been 'weaponised'. If deviance can be effectively appended to stigma, then the austerity of neoliberalism that seeks to blame and punish the vulnerable might obtain sufficient purchase to open the door to further welfare cuts and sell-offs and to enhanced capital accumulation. Drawing on the earlier discussion, and in particular on Table 6.2, if the stigmatised can be portrayed as deviants, then the category of 'losers' can be supplemented as 'rejects' are recast as 'abjects'. And abjects are both completely beyond the pale and deserving of their lot and their misery. The weaponising of stigma allows for the state's abandonment of whole segments of the population.

There is much that is Victorian in the newfound propensity to blame the poor and vulnerable for their poverty and vulnerability. As many have said, it smacks of long abandoned 'poor laws'. Given the opening fractures in British society, the weaponising of stigma has a special resonance. A series of populist, anti-establishment, nationalist – and some are suggesting 'proto-fascist' – risings in Britain, the USA and much of Europe have culminated, respectively, in 'Brexit', the election of Trump and far-right electoral threats. In the next chapter, focusing on transformation, I shall précis a class analysis of this; but it is sufficient for now to note that a backlash against the calculated class- and command-based demonisation of segments of the working class, embracing the weaponising of stigma, contributes significantly to the explanation of Brexit, Trump and the popularity of the likes of Le Pen.

The fractured society and health inequalities

In previous chapters, I developed the thesis that financial capitalism's principal feature, a refreshed and reinvigorated class/command dynamic, is pivotal for a credible sociology of health inequalities. In this chapter I have broadened the account to suggest that financial capitalism has delivered a fractured society in Britain (and indeed elsewhere). Fissures that have become fractures include hidden forms of system-cum-social disintegration that threaten the implosion of capitalism itself, largely unacknowledged class divisions and polarisation, a digitalised form of McDonaldisation that exploits and oppresses consumers in the name of bespoke free choice, a surfeit of cultural liquidity leaking its way into the lifeworld, clandestine network domination via superhubs and a political deployment of shame and blame to 'other' and subdue disadvantaged people lacking the wherewithal to fight back. These fractures promise sharp, short-term benefits for the capital executive and its class and political allies *even as they whisper 'risk'*.

What ramifications do these dimensions of a fractured society hold for health and health inequalities? The 21 theses that follow are an attempt to draw together heterogeneous, loose threads:

1 first among the social mechanisms responsible for health inequalities in post-1970s financial capitalism is the class/command dynamic;
2 this dynamic attributes primary causal responsibility for health inequalities to the capitalist executive in general, and the superhub capital monopolists in particular;
3 health inequalities are an unintended consequence of the strategic decision-making of this mere fraction of the 1% identified and chastised by Occupy (hence the GBH);

4 the media of enactment of the GBH are a discrete set of asset flows, understood objectively but also impacting subjectively (in line with people's reference groups);

5 meso or middle-rage theories are critical and under-represented, witness Seigrist's model of effort-reward imbalance, Goldthorpe's risk aversion model, plus those of ego adjustment and activity reinforcement outlined earlier;

6 Seigrist's model helps reinforce deepening inequalities as the rich or affluent and powerful or influential experience and perceive rewards for their efforts while those lacking these advantages do not (with the health sequelae Seigrist charts);

7 Goldthorpe's model is salient in so far as working-class and precarious middle-class personnel and families make their priority consolidation and the avoidance of risk-taking out of a fear of further deterioration, a process akin, most notably in the working class, to a slippage into vulnerable fractured reflexivity;

8 the ego adjustment model speaks of a parallel tendency, namely, for individuals to commit to narrative rationales (or rationalisations) that underwrite (render understandable and positive) perceptions and actions emanating from their social positioning, thus re-affirming the status quo;

9 the activity reinforcement model also favours reconciliation to the status quo, this time via a familiarity of day-to-day repetition associated with people's status and role sets that translates into predictable behaviours and is beyond the conscious reach of ego adjustment;

10 the more likely people with (clusters of) those weak asset flows known to be pertinent for health and longevity, the more likely they are to be reconciled or resigned to, or show passivity toward, neoliberal ideology, and the less likely they are to act individually or collectively to promote advantageous change;

11 the short-term prospects are for a deepening of health inequalities;

12 a strong case can be made that financial capitalism is spiralling out of control and imploding, with little effective opposition and, relatedly, checks and balances and effective crisis management compromised;

13 the possibility of an imminent crisis of legitimation remains;

14 the cultural shift from grand to petit narratives and current excess of cultural liquidity undermine narrative opposition to the neoliberal status quo;

15 there has been a weaponising of stigma as the largely working-class disadvantaged and vulnerable ('abjects') have been targeted for austerity cuts;

16 the McDonaldised digitalisation of health (self-)management and care is a double-edged sword, contributing more to capitalist executive investors and their allies than to people-as-patients;

17 health policy and health care remain at the mercy of the class/command dynamic, with the prospect of damage apparently too deep to rectify;

18 a populist trend towards the right of the political spectrum threatens a regressive evocation of a US-like abandonment of universal health care

of which the Cameron-to-May privatisation/commodification of health care in England/Wales is witness;

19 for all this prognostic gloom, the volitivity and likely implosion of capitalism, plus climate change, global migration and the post-Bexit, Trump and proto-fascist initiatives, afford *some* prospects for a subversive politics;

20 professional and policy sociologies have largely vacated this Bourdieu-like 'field', with critical and public sociologies not making good the deficit;

21 we as sociologists owe it to our discipline and ourselves to engage via foresight and action initiatives.

So, how might these theses be further clarified and, crucially, what collective, agential, transformative potential might survive them? These are the questions addressed in the opening sections of the next chapter. The final chapter then amounts to a manifesto for a sociology fit for purpose, while the concluding paragraphs sketch a research programme for a sociology of health and health inequalities. It is a programme that I regard as vital but that some of my colleagues in sociology and companion disciplines will doubtless see as scandalous and likely to bring us all into disrepute.

7 Transformative politics and change

Bhaskar (2016: 120) writes:

> focusing on social analysis, absence has a remarkable diagnostic value. Looking at a social situation and asking what is *not* there, what is missing, will often give the researcher an invaluable insight into how the situation needs to change and/or how it will change.

So, what to do? This chapter faces up to the parameters for purposive collective change that directly or indirectly address the (mal)distribution of health. Furthermore, I agree with Streeck's (2016) general view that sociology has lost its way in so far as it has come to neglect 'economic sociology', a core component of classical sociology. The issues I have touched on here, and that are *absolutely key* for a tenable macro- to meso- to micro-sociology of health and health inequalities, are mostly 'absent' from extant efforts, as are evidence-based sketches of alternative policies, institutions and arrangements. Bhaskar's power 2 relations are alluded to, then side-stepped.

First, the intricate complexity of accounting for change should be accented. It is a programme that spans strata and must allow for emergence and dialectics even as it turns its back on inter-stratum reducibility. Bhaskar (2016: 56) reminds us too that social science can operate at different 'levels of scale'. Thus:

- *sub-individual*, psychological level, including the Freudian unconscious and that of our ordinary attributions of motives and reasons for action;
- *individual* or biographical level, typically adopted by novelists but also argued by some (such as Sartre), not just individualists, to be the most important in the social sciences;
- *micro-level* studied for example by ethnomethodologists, concerned with such issues as turn-taking in conversation or how we avoid bumping into each other on the pavement;
- *meso-level* at which we might be concerned with the relations between functional roles, such as capitalist and worker or politician and citizen;

- *macro-level*, oriented to understanding the functioning of whole sectors of society, such as the British economy;
- *mega-level*, concerned with the tracing and analysis of trajectories of whole traditions or formations, such as feudalism or contemporary Islamic fundamentalism; and
- *planetary* (or *cosmological*) level, at which we are concerned with the planet (or cosmos) as a whole, as for example in Immanuel Wallerstein's world-systems theory. This level may also be extended to cover the whole *geo-history* of humanity or the planet, and so on.

Bhaskar has social science rather than sociology in mind here. It is axiomatic nevertheless that: (a) sociology can in principal input into each of these seven levels of scale, and (b) the argument being compiled in the present volume is modest and limited, focusing as it does on the meso-, macro- and mega-levels (with an occasional nod to the micro-level).

Bhaskar (2016: 102) preserves an important role also for critical discourse analysis, that is, 'the analysis of value-impregnated and ideologically saturated discourse, relating such discourse back to its conditions of production in such a way as to bring out the practical implications and presuppositions of the discourse'. Such discourse involves power 2 relations.

In this chapter, I begin by reiterating and developing an analysis of the *context* – the fractured society of financial capitalism – in which transformative change must occur. In the second section, Archer's analysis of reflexivity is mined again, this time to proffer an ideal type of likely individual agents of transformation, the *dedicated meta-reflexives*. This dimension of agency is contextualised in terms of possible structural and cultural precipitants of change. Third, I consider *future scenarios* – Bhaskar (2016: 93) writes of 'concrete utopias' – this time drawing in particular on the pioneering work of Urry (2016). The fourth section samples Mason's (2015) package of economic reforms and the notion of 'permanent reform'.

The end of capitalism?

Capitalism has often been said to be in a terminal state. Most recently, the global financial crisis of 2008–2009 was widely pronounced to be fatal, and yet Streeck's (2016) new book has a cautious title, *How Will Capitalism End?* His central thesis, however, is more audacious. It is that we are currently living in an 'interregnum', with financial capitalism attempting suicide and no sign of either an effective intervention or any ready-made successor. Streeck's (2016: 232) account might be read as an eloquent formulation of the class/command dynamic:

> … the decline of post-war pacified capitalism must primarily be attributed to endogenous subversion and erosion of an institutional framework that had become suboptimal for capital accumulation, rather than …

to the frivolous fancies of neoliberal economists and misled politicians. Post-war democratic capitalism was fragile from its beginning – it only looked stable due to extraordinary political circumstances and the studied optimism of political leaders after the end of the war. In fact it could never hope to last longer than, in historical terms, a very short period. When it began to decay in the 1970s, it was because of the helplessness of democratic politics, organized at and confined to the level of nation states, against capitalism's new international opportunities for evading the social constraints that had by the 1970s landed it in an increasingly uncomfortable profit squeeze. For a time, the dependence of politics and political success under democratic capitalism on uninterrupted capital accumulation – or in the technocratic language of standard economics: on economic growth – led inevitably optimistic politicians to place their hopes on riding the tiger and jump on the historical bandwagon towards liberalization and deregulation until the re-formed capitalist economic regime almost crashed as a result of its unfettered progress.

One more complementary quotation from Streeck (2016: 233) is warranted:

> Capitalism … is 'always embedded' in that it takes place in a society, subject to social constraints and opportunities. Also, capitalism in an important sense depends on remaining so embedded as it thrives on the rule of law, mutual trust, normative coordination and institutionalized cooperation, creative intelligence and the like. Nevertheless, and at the same time, capitalist actors always struggle to escape from their social containment and free themselves from obligations and controls. Ideas of solidarity and institutions of social regulation are as a result at a permanent risk of erosion, with capitalist patterns of action spreading like cancer in the body social even though capitalism as such, pure and simple and liberated from social constraints, cannot exist. In this sense capitalism feeds parasitically on the society that it inhabits or befalls, with its expansion ultimately amounting to its self-destruction unless checked by social and political opposition. Sometimes, as in the neoliberal era, the capitalist advance may capture the very politics that should contain it for its own good, and turn it into a vehicle of its own self-destructive progress …

I would add at this point, pace C Wright Mills, that the interests of core actors within the capitalist executive and the political or power elite have come to *overlap*.

Streeck's argument that financial capitalism is imploding, in the process occasioning what I call societal fracturing, rests on a number of companion trends or, using critical realist terms, tendencies. He positively cites Marx on capitalism's contradictions and its propensity to induce fractures. In his view, without opposition capitalism will destroy itself: and in financial capitalism, it is suffering from an overdose of itself. He highlights a quintet of telling 'disorders': (a) stagnation, (b) oligarchic redistribution, (c) the plundering of the public domain, (d) corruption and (e) global anarchy.

Stagnation theories often approximate to Marxist theories of underconsumption. Although those comprising the governing oligarchy seem to be adapting to low or no growth (excepting of course high profits in the financial sector, attained via speculative trading with cheap monies on offer from central banks), 'bubbles are waiting to burst'. This is likely to end as 'a struggle for survival', 'a battle of all against all, punctured by occasional panics and with the playing of endgames becoming a popular pastime' (Streeck, 2016: 67).

With reference to oligarchic redistribution, there is no immediate prospect of the present redistribution from poor to rich citizens, with all its ramifications for health, longevity and health care, being stalled, let alone reversed. As much was anticipated 'in the infamous "plutonomy" memorandum distributed by Citibank in 2005 and 2006 to a select circle of its richest clients, to assure them that their prosperity no longer depended on that of wage earners' (Streeck, 2016: 68).

The governing oligarchy is enriching itself by 'plundering' (via underfunding and privatisation), ultimately to its own detriment. Witness the systematic destruction of the NHS. But also, capitalist lemmings to the clifftop. 'Even before 2008, it was generally taken for granted that the fiscal crisis of the post-war state had to be resolved by lowering spending instead of raising taxes, especially on the rich. Consolidation of public finances by way of austerity was and is being imposed on societies even though it is likely to depress growth' (Streeck, 2016: 69).

And what of corruption? Unsparingly, Streeck pinpoints the financial sector, 'ugly' profiteering (e.g. asset stripping on an industrial scale), moral decline and public cynicism (see also Standing, 2016). Whilst Weber once took pains to distinguish between capitalism and greed, they have become increasingly synonymous; and greed has, in turn, become synonymous with corruption.

Streeck's last disorder is global anarchy. Global capitalism needs a centre to secure its periphery, Streeck claims, echoing Wallerstein. This role was performed by Britain up to the 1920s and, after a period of 'chaos', by the USA from 1945 to the 1970s (Scambler & Scambler, 2013). The USA can no longer fulfil this role, and the dollar's function as an international reserve currency is uncertain. The USA is no longer a global guarantor or 'enforcer'.

Capitalism, Streeck rightly concludes, is in a critical condition; but it does not follow, as he accepts, that a replacement regime is in the wings. For the record, he mounts an 'unfashionable' argument for socialism, to which I return later; that is as maybe. But to whom might we realistically look as agents of change?

Archer, dedicated meta-reflexives and triggers for change

(a) Dedicated meta-reflexives

So how, and by means of what agency, might transformative change towards socialism or elsewhere be accomplished? After all, it is now more anachronism than platitude within sociological circles that people have beliefs, values and attitudes that owe more to their natal or involuntary placement in society than to the exercise of agency. As has been made plain, however, Bhaskar and Archer acknowledge as much but yet allow for the transformative power of agency. Resistance to the neoliberal status quo necessarily involves countering, subverting and ultimately undermining the global/national/local potency of ideology, in the present the ideology of neoliberalism. And the accumulated evidence of the post-welfare-statist decades leads ineluctably to the conclusion that health inequalities in the UK and elsewhere cannot be addressed effectively by Popperian 'piecemeal social engineering': meaningful resistance *necessarily* reaches deep down into generative social mechanisms, be they of structure, culture *or agency*. The class/command dynamic that characterises the present represents the key and overriding structural input into health inequalities/inequities. But what of the potentially transformative power of agency?

For Archer, meta-reflexives, oriented by values, are characterised by 'contextual incongruity', which denotes an incongruity between dreams and aspirations and contextual factors that obstruct their realization. But not all dreams and hopes fade away, and those organizers and leaders of resistance to neoliberal ideology might be said to represent a subset of meta-reflexives whose value-driven commitments become central to identity for self and others and transmute into lifelong advocacy on behalf of the 'community as a whole'. I call them *dedicated meta-reflexives.*

These putative activists might superficially appear to resemble the contingent of focused autonomous reflexives characterised earlier; but Archer separates them unambiguously. While the focused autonomous reflexives are almost entirely instrumental, strategically, single-mindedly and ruthlessly oriented to the pursuit of their own interests, the dedicated meta-reflexives are value, other- and community- or 'third sector'-oriented. As Archer (2007b) shows, the:

> ... meta-reflexive concern for 'community', despite its varied meanings, is light years removed from both the communicative reflexives' preoccupation with their own micro-life worlds and the autonomous reflexives' use of the locality as a place for out-sourcing and paid access to selected facilities ... what unites (meta-reflexives) is not a burgeoning communitarianism, but rather a common belief that social problems will not yield to individualistic incentives or to centralized political interventions.

Marmot often cites Neruda's injunction to 'rise up with me against the organization of misery', a plea he regards as an international rather than national or local call to arms. There is a question here of the degree of commitment to 'making a difference'. Terry Eagleton (2011) writes:

> reform is vital; but sooner or later you will hit a point where the system refuses to give way, and for Marxism this is known as the social relations of production. Or, in less polite technical language, a dominant class which controls the material resources and is markedly reluctant to hand them over. It is only then that a decisive choice between reform and revolution looms up.

In a neoliberal era, Marmot has fought nobly but mostly unavailingly. If he and sociologists of health inequalities are (in a Hegelian sense) 'serious', then there will have to be a sociological reckoning with the contradictions of capitalism and the likes of transnational and national relations of class and command, a step far beyond an abstruse, academic fascination with socio-economic group/status (SEG/S), the social gradient and health. The SEG/S and its association with health cannot be explained sociologically in the absence of a more comprehensive theory of social class and class struggle.

Key protagonists in such a struggle are presented here as *dedicated meta-reflexives* (Scambler, 2012b). Given the low visibility of class politics in the neoliberal era, dedicated meta-reflexives are unlikely to see themselves, or be seen by others, as class warriors engaged in an ongoing struggle. They are more likely to be the issue of a heterogeneous array of 'mobilizing potentials'. Some of their number, whether campaigning against the hike in student fees, the abolition of the Education Maintenance Allowance or the Health and Social Care Bill, might be paid up members of an anti-capitalist 'movement of movements', but others are manifestly not. The characteristics of this subtype of meta-reflexives might be summarised as follows:

(a) Impulse to solidarity

Picking up on Archer's narrative, dedicated meta-reflexives are oriented to community. In Habermasian terms, their natural mode of relating is communicative rather than strategic. Their actions are informed by values of sociality, favouring norms of reciprocity.

(b) System immunity

Activists falling within the category of dedicated meta-reflexive have strong ego-defences, allowing them to have enduring lifeworld rather than system ambition. Their aspirations are unlikely to be easily undone by, Habermas again, the 'steering media' of the economy or state, that is, money or power.

(c) A predilection to optimism

Optimism of the will subduing pessimism of the intellect is likely to be on the calling cards of dedicated meta-reflexives. These are disciples of Gramsci, refusing not to act against the odds. They do not just have 'system immunity' but are committed to better futures.

(d) Visionary insight

However embryonic, the dedicated meta-reflexive envisages a future that improves on past and present, and does so for the 'community as a whole' rather than a discrete (wealthy, powerful) segment (like the CCE/PE). Their vision belongs within Giddens' category of 'utopian realism'.

(e) Therapeutic orientation

Dedicated meta-reflexives 'care' in ways often antipathetic to instrumental or strategic action. Their challenge is Lenin's and is around Hegel's notion of 'seriousness'.

(e) Action commitment

It is in their predisposition to act, to intervene, to make a difference, that the dedicated meta-reflexives' therapeutic orientation is leavened by engagement. There may be a tension here, however, between actions aimed at *consensus* and actions aimed at *outcome*. Which do dedicated meta-reflexives privilege, representing the communities in which they participate or securing benefits on their behalf? Or is it necessary to choose? Castells (2012) suggests that contemporary movements are more consensual than their predecessors.

The same caveats apply as did to the ideal types of focused autonomous and vulnerable fractured reflexives advanced earlier. There is no implication that dedicated meta-reflexivity precisely matches empirical cases, is permanent or spans all status- and role-sets. The extent of what is claimed is that this is one way in which agency is socially structured without being socially determined, and for which there is a measure of substantive support. Collins et al. (2015) have suggested it might reflect my/sociologists' (and maybe metropolitan liberals' (Winlow et al., 2017)) sense of self-worth and self-engagement, which is a possibility yet to be tested.

(b) Triggers for change

If Streeck is correct in announcing a spiralling implosion of capitalism in its post-1970s financial guise, and this can credibly be linked to the fracturing of society, then it would seem that the preconditions exist for societal transformation. As ever, it is a tale of swings and roundabouts: there are enabling and constraining forces at work. I shall list the constraining factors first:

- financial capitalism remains at full throttle, for all that it now seems 'out of control';
- its contradictions and generative mechanisms are largely invisible;
- their 'invisibility' owes much to the 'there is no alternative' (TINA) ideology that most benefits the capitalist executive and its new and old middle-class allies and co-optees;
- it has become profoundly difficult to articulate a convincing 'grand narrative' in opposition to the TINA ideology;
- the lack of an alternative vision for the future has its origins in: (a) a class/state underwriting of TINA and (b) a structural/cultural shift to postmodern or relativised 'petit narratives';
- the result of this shift is that angry and frustrated citizens-cum-consumers are clearer about what they oppose than they are about alternative and better futures;
- the dissolution of the input of (subjective) class consciousness into identity-formation has robbed the 'angry and frustrated' of the prime mechanism of resistance to financial capitalism and the healing of the multiple fractures the capitalist executive has facilitated or otherwise welcomed and reinforced;
- in Britain and in many other western countries, former left-of-centre or social democratic political parties have: (a) drifted to the right in line with TINA and/or (b) failed, albeit in inauspicious circumstances, to deliver a vision of an alternative and better future;
- this structural/cultural 'vacuum' has witnessed a resurgence of right-wing populism, in Britain extending beyond UKIP and Brexit to encompass proto-fascist activism;
- this protest of the angry and frustrated has precipitated a reasonable and emotional abandonment of the Labour Party in its former industrial-era strongholds in the Midlands and the North, with many votes switching to UKIP;
- at the time of writing, Corbyn's contested, left-of-centre leadership of the Labour Party is seeking to recapture this lost ground;
- recalling Miliband's (1961) thinking *even prior to the onset of financial capitalism*, there seems little or no prospect of change engineered piecemeal via the state institutions of 'parliamentary capitalism'.

So what of the enabling thrust? Here is my counter-list to a powerful series of constraints:

- if the thesis of capitalism's chickens belatedly coming home to roost is viable, and I think it is, then the resultant turmoil offers up (left-wing) opportunity as well as (right-wing) hazard;
- the anger and frustration emergent from a disillusion with the establishment, the Westminster Bubble, political careerism and corruption and continued neglect by London-centric regimes has potential to fuel a left- rather than a right-oriented populism;

- although the capitalist executive and the state representatives it purchased survived the financial crisis of 2008–2009 (*and some*), the conditions that led to that crisis persist, meaning that a new crisis and one of legitimation is still on the cards;
- the most likely 'unmanageable' crisis maybe what Habermas (1975) calls a 'rationality crisis', whereby the state fails to deliver economically to significant segments of the electorate;
- it is improbable that a rationality crisis will be generated or occur in the absence of an (unpredictable) 'triggering episode';
- another critical precondition is a resonating 'narrative' projecting a better, achievable future;
- despite the popularity of its policy programme, the Labour Party conspicuously lacked such a narrative in the run-up to the 2015 general election, though Corbyn's narrative is stronger and more coherent;
- likely sources for such a narrative, capturing and giving voice to the kind of anger and frustration that occurred when the metropolitan police twice shot Mark Duggan in dubious circumstances on 4 August 2011, are extra-parliamentary and range from campaign-specific through rights-based and (new) social movement to workplace or welfare activism (Scambler & Kelleher, 2006);
- a likely precondition for effective opposition is nevertheless *class-based collective action*, which, given the deep-cut salience of real (objective) class relations in financial capitalism, is always lurking;
- working-class engagement is the prepotent challenge.

Out of the changes taking place within our fractured society, which have been characterised as techtonic, new futures might emerge. If only sociology were predictive! But then again, capitalism has outlived many previous crises of legitimation.

Future studies

'Future studies' has acquired a momentum of its own. Moreover, it holds the promise of visions of alternate social worlds and institutions. Urry (2016) underlines the generally slow pace of deep, structural change. Archer's morphogenetic cycles noted in Chapter 4, with structural conditioning shaping social interaction and leading, ultimately, to structural elaboration, is a time-consuming process. Urry cites the historian Braudel in this connection but might equally have called to mind Elias's (1939) sociology of the 'civilising process'. He quotes Raymond Williams (1977: 132) on the compelling idea of 'structures of feeling':

> 'feeling' is chosen to emphasize a distinction from more formal concepts of 'world view' or 'ideology'. It is not only that we must go beyond formally held and systematic beliefs ... we are concerned with meanings and values as they are actively lived and felt ... not feeling against

thought, but thought as felt and feeling as thought: practical consciousness of a present kind, in a living and interrelating continuity. We are
then defining these elements as a 'structure': as a set, with specific internal relations, at once interlocking and in tension.

Urry applies Williams's thinking to the transition to and impact of financial
capitalism, suggesting that 'a striking change of the structure of feeling or
Zeitgeist within the rich North emerged after the optimism of the roaring
1990s was blown away. This long-term "catastrophism" within much social
and scientific thought can be seen in many texts dating from 2003 onwards'
(Urry, 2016: 35).

Recent versions of catastrophism address the broad – in Bhaskar's terms
planetary or cosmological – issue of climate change, and Urry, drawing
loosely on Luhmann's systems theory and complexity theory, devotes much
of his discussion to this literature. It is a sense of catastrophe beyond that of
financial capitalism in crisis. To the notion of societal change, occasioned
by insinuating climate change, might be appended that already underway
as a result of new patterns of mass migration prompted by incipient climate
change as well as by war and economic hardship. The focus here, however,
is necessarily more parochial (though it is recognised that planetary/cosmo-
logical shifts threaten even those societies like Britain that suffer least from
the 'boomerang effects' of the risks that Beck (1982) highlighted a generation ago. For all the emphasis on contemporary processes of globalisation,
the rich societies comprising the Occident have broken away into relatively
protected and 'fortified' enclaves, othering the (semi- and peripheral) wild
zones outside their boundaries, even as – courtesy of their globalised, nomadic and post-national capitalist executives – they exploit them. 'Bleak impoverished societies face regular breakdowns of civil order and a crippling
incapacity to resolve system crises. Their populations regularly try to jump
over offshored barriers in order to enter the safe zones (with increasing numbers dying en route)' (Urry, 2016: 50–51).

The future is not sitting there awaiting recognition. Urry recalls Buckmin-
ster Fuller's assertion that 'you never change anything by fighting the existing reality. To change something, build a new model that makes the existing
model obsolete' (Urry, 2016: 78). As someone versed in dialectical realism
might say, think your way into the immense ocean of absence rather than react
to the ripple of presence. Move beyond dystopias to utopias. The capacity to
think futures, Bauman (1976: 13) once said, is emancipatory: 'the presence of
a utopia, the ability to think of alternative solutions to the festering problems
of the present, may be seen therefore as a necessary condition of historical
change.' Urry (2016: 97) refers in this context to 'scenario building': 'scenario
development involves establishing a characterisation of the economy or society for a future year in the light of known trends, the main sources of change
and the likely patterns of economic and social life.' This invites input outside
of sociology of course, but if my earlier commendation of foresight sociology
has any purchase at all, it is also an acute challenge to sociology.

Unhappily, Urry did not directly broach issues of health and health inequalities. His comments not only on climate change but on a post-car society are instructive however (and a matter of some relevance to public health). The health, environmental and energy consequences of car usage, he argued (Urry, 2016: 134–135), have been recognised; business-as-usual is no longer an uncontested option; experimentation in relation to alternative design, fuel types and charging systems by small- and medium-sized enterprises, NGOs, city governments and transnational corporations is well underway; urban design too is adapting to car future restraint; uncertainties around the future of supply of oil and use of fossil fuels are being addressed; it is being recognised that cities with less car-based movement are associated with higher levels of wellbeing for residents and visitors; there has already been some reduction in car use in car-dependent societies, including decreasing numbers of young drivers and a growth in car-free times and zones in cities; and there is evidence in some countries that millennials prefer smartphones and other forms of high-tech accessories to cars. Unsurprisingly, Urry accepts that the forces acting against the realisation of alternatives to car usage nevertheless remain strong.

In line with the presentation of the revised class/command dynamic of financial capitalism advanced here, Urry (2016: 173) writes:

> contemporary capitalism is transformed into a significantly untaxed, ungovernable and out-of-control financial capitalism. The scale of finance is enormous and works more like gambling. Its growth and domination of the industrial economy, as well as of the physical environment, has magnified economic, social and property inequalities in most countries ... Especially significant here are the multiple processes of offshoring: the movement of resources, practices, people and monies from territory to territory and hiding them. It involves evading rules, laws, taxes, regulations or norms ... In particular, there has been an astonishing growth in the movement of finance and wealth through the world's sixty to seventy tax havens, representing close to one-third of all contemporary societies ... Tax havens are places of low taxes, wealth management, deregulation and secrecy, and became absolutely core to the world economy, as exchange and related controls were removed from the 1970s onwards.

Bearing in mind the empirical credibility, even obviousness, of the GBH, where in the contemporary sociology of health inequalities are the analyses of the causal role of the likes of tax havens, let alone the spelling out of alternative socio-economic, public health and health care policies allied to the concept of a foresight sociology?

Future scenarios and 'permanent reform'

Capitalism's days may or may not be numbered. Streeck maintains that the die is likely cast, but it is always wise to be wary given the record of obduracy of this hoary, centuries-old socio-economic system. As Urry discusses, there exist numerous fictitious portrayals of apocalyptic social collapse and post-capitalist formations, plus some drawing on established research. I will not rehearse these again (see Urry, 2016: Chapter 2). Instead I will outline in some detail and comment on one effort of diagnosis and prognosis, Mason's *Postcapitalism: A Guide to Our Future*, 2015. Mason arrives at a conclusion compatible with Streeck's, if by a circuitous route. What is of special interest here, however, is his pinpointing and advocacy of remedies, together with their salience for health and the 'tackling' of health inequalities. He offers five ways of translating his analysis into a 'project' offering five principals of transition.

(1) Understand the limitations of human will-power

Confronted by a complex, fragile (and to use my own term, 'fractured) system, there are limits to people's capacity to see and act clearly and with intent and stamina. The moral, Mason suggests, is to pilot and test policy change before laying it out on a national scale. He cites the murdered Soviet economist Preobrazhensky (1964: 55), who called for 'an extremely complex and ramified nervous system of social foresight and planned guidance'. While all the Soviet's had was command, control and a bureaucratic hierarchy, Mason continues, we have networks. Networks carry greater potential for change, but only if the complexity and fragility of our highly differentiated contemporary societies are respected.

(2) Ecological sustainability

We can expect to be 'hit' by the likes of short-term localised energy shortages over the next decade, ageing and migration challenges over the next 30 years and the catastrophic outcomes of climate change not long after that.

(3) The transition is not just about economics

The transition to postcapitalism must be seen as *human* rather than (merely) economic: 'the new kinds of people being created by networked economies come with new insecurities and new priorities' (Mason, 2015: 267). New forms of democracy will be needed to arbitrate between competing models and alternative possibilities.

(4) Attack the problem from all angles

The networked society is not as constrained as its predecessors. Swarms of individuals can be effective agents of change as they cross the boundaries of states, corporations and political parties. The focus at present tends to be on experimental, small-scale projects, for example credit unions. This focus must be broadened 'so that solutions can be found through a mixture of small-scale experiment, proven models that can be scaled up and top-down action by states ... So if the solution in finance is to create a diverse, socialised banking system, then setting up a credit union attacks the problem from one direction, outlawing certain forms of speculation attacks it from another, while changing our own financial behaviour attacks it from still another angle' (Mason, 2015: 267–268).

(5) Maximise the power of information

The aggregated data comprising much of our lives will in the immanent future capture citizen-cum-consumers' weekly diet, body mass and heart rate, and will constitute an influential 'social technology' in and of itself. It will be a new 'social machine'. It will have the capacity to optimise resources but also, by 'socializing knowledge', to amplify the results of collective action: it holds the prospect of going beyond a decentralisation of control towards 'collaborative control':

> for example, in epidemiology the focus is now on breaking the feedback loops that create poverty, anger, stress, atomised families and ill-health. Efforts to map these problems and mitigate them constitute the cutting edge of social medicine. How much more powerful would that medicine be if the poverty and disease that blight poor communities could be mapped, understood and collaboratively dismantled in realtime – with the micro-level participation of those affected?
>
> (Mason, 2015: 269)

Laying out basic principles and formulating policy are different things. Mason is circumspect. He sets out four 'top level aims' for a postcapitalist regimen, which I sketch in Table 7.1. But he offers more. We must, he advises, create a global network to actively, openly and 'accessibly' *simulate* the long-term transition beyond capitalism. We must also 'switch off the neoliberal privatisation machine'. The state's *neutrality* re-capitalism is a myth: 'it typically deregulates finance, forces government to outsource services and allows public healthcare, education and transport to become shoddy, driving people to privatise services' (Mason, 2015: 273). The state must reshape markets in favour of sustainable, collaborative and socially just outcomes. It must plan and 'own' the agenda for change, most urgently in relation to debt. It would be sensible, he claims,

> to combine controlled debt write-offs with a ten- to fifteen-year global policy of 'financial repression': that is, to stimulate inflation, hold interest rates lower than the inflation rate, remove people's ability to move money into non-financial investments or offshore, and thus inflate away the debts, writing off the part that remained.
>
> (Mason, 2015: 275)

Table 7.1 Mason's Key Goals for a Postcapitalist Project

- Rapidly reduce carbon emissions so that the world warms by two degrees Celsius by 2050, which might prevent an energy crisis and mitigate the chaos promised by climate events;
- Stabilise the financial system before 2050 by socialising it, so that ageing populations, climate change and debt do not combine to detonate a new boom-bust cycle and destroy the world economy;
- Deliver high levels of material prosperity and wellbeing to the majority of the 99%, primarily by prioritising information-rich technologies to solve major social challenges, such as ill health, welfare dependency, sexual exploitation and deficient education;
- Gear technology towards the reduction of 'necessary work' to promote a rapid transition to an automated economy (so that work becomes 'voluntary, basic commoditied and public services are free, and economic management becomes first and foremost an issue of energy and resources, not capital and labour.

Source: Adapted from Mason (2015).

Collaborative businesses have the potential to pave the way for positive change, that is, if they go beyond existing co-op models to give rise to a legal framework allowing for 'a real, collaborative form of production or consumption, with clear social outcomes' (Mason, 2015: 276). There is no need to fetishise non-profit making, but the tax system should be rejigged: (a) to reward the creation of non-profits and collaborative production and (b) to make it hard to form low-wage businesses but easy to form living-wage ones. Large corporations would need to be constrained by law and regulation:

> if we legally empowered the workforces of global corporations with strong employment rights, their owners would be forced to promote high-wage, high-growth, high-technology economic models, instead of the opposite. The low-wage, low-skill and low-quality corporations that have flourished since the 1990s exist only because the space for them was ruthlessly carved out by the state
>
> (Mason, 2015: 277)

Models no less radical emerged in the past in the teeth of opposition from plantation owners and factory bosses. Postcapitalism must be 'regularised'.

The creation of monopolies to resist falling prices is a vital device or 'defence reflex' against postcapitalism. Mason argues that monopolies should be outlawed whenever possible and price fixing regulated. Public ownership should be the default option when it is impractical to forego monopolies. The underlying goal would be to cheapen the cost of basic necessities. True public provision of water, energy, housing, transport, health care, telecoms infrastructure and education would be a compelling strategic act of redistribution. 'The state, the corporate sector and public corporations could be made to pursue radically different ends with relatively low-cost changes to regulation, underpinned by a radical commitment to shrink debt' (Mason, 2015: 278).

The postcapitalist society Mason envisages is not based on command planning. There would be no need for the abolition of markets by diktat. Instead, he commends a position in which *profit derives from entrepreneurship, not rent*. Patents and intellectual property should taper away quickly (drug licences already expire after 20 years). Governments might insist that the results of state-funded research should be effectively free at the point of use, shifting everything delivered via public funding into a Habermasian public sphere and, thereby, nudging the balance of intellectual property from private into common usage. In the field of energy in particular, Mason argues, it is imperative to swiftly suppress market forces because of climate change: the state should assume ownership and control of the energy distribution grid, plus all big carbon-based suppliers of energy. Renewable technologies should be subsidised, when possible in private companies. Household use of energy should be eased into efficient usage. Space, as ever, must be left for innovation. 'Once information technology pervades the physical world, every innovation brings us closer to the world of zero necessary work' (Mason, 2015: 280).

Mason also advocates the 'socialization' of the financial system. Moreover, if the risks associated with financial capitalism are to be socialised, the rewards should be too. The triad of measures he proposes are summarised in Table 7.2. He admits that these are short-term measures that fall short of a recipe for a postcapitalist financial system. Also required is credit creation and an expanded money supply to mediate the debt pile that is strangling growth. But credit creation only works if it prompts the market sector to grow (so the borrower can repay the loan with interest). The state, via the central bank, would have to step in to underwrite this process. The overriding aim, however, would not be to achieve some kind of 'steady state capitalism' but to ease the way to postcapitalism.

Mason goes on to advocate a universal basic income guaranteed by the state (a project since being piloted outside of Britain; see Standing, 2017). He sees its purpose as radical: (a) to make formal the separation of work and wages and (b) to subsidise the transition to 'a shorter working week, or day, or life' (Mason, 2015; 284). It would in effect socialise the costs of automation:

> the idea is simple: everybody of working age gets an unconditional basic income from the state, funded from taxation, and this replaces unemployment benefit. Other forms of needs-based welfare – such as family, disability or child payments – would continue to exist, but would be smaller top-ups to the basic income.
>
> (Mason, 2015: 284)

The phenomenon of automation was mentioned earlier. Automation *under neoliberalism* would entail an expansion of 'precarity'. But a basic income would allow for time-outs and rethinks (Standing, 2017). In isolation from 'an overall transition project' it would be overly costly and would fail; but it has a strong potential. Its promotion recognises that there are, and will

Table 7.2 Measures to Socialise the Financial System

1   Nationalise the central bank, setting it a target for sustainable growth and an inflation target designed to facilitate: (a) 'a socially just form of financial repression' and (b) 'a controlled write-down of the massive debt overhang'. The inevitable antagonism might be dissipated 'if a systemic economy did this'. A sustainability target, modelled against climatic, demographic and social impact, would be critical. The monetary policy of the central bank should become explicit, transparent and under political control.
2   Restructure the banking system to yield a mix of utilities earning capped profit rates, non-profit local and regional banks, credit unions and peer-to peer lenders and a comprehensive state-owned provider of financial services. The state would be lender of last resort to these banks.
3   Leave a regulated space for 'complex' financial activities, which would allow for the sector's return to a historical role of efficiently allocating resources between firms, savers, lenders and so on. This role would be buttressed by strict criminal enforcement as well as professional codes in banking, accountancy and law. The overriding principle would be to reward innovation whilst discouraging and penalising rent-seeking behaviour. It would be a breach of professional ethics for example for a chartered accountant or qualified lawyer to propose a tax avoidance scheme, or for a hedge fund to store uranium in a warehouse to drive its spot price higher. In countries like Britain, governments should offer a deal whereby, in return for 'coming clearly and transparently onshore', some limited lender of last resort facilities should be made available to remaining high-risk, profit-oriented finance firms. Those declining to come onshore 'would be treated as the financial equivalent of Al-Qaeda'.

Source: Adapted from Mason (2015).

increasingly be, too few work hours to go round, so there is a need to inject 'liquidity' into the mechanisms that allocate them. A basic income would remove the stigma, and the compounding deviance, of not working and would stack the labour market in favour of the higher-paying job and the higher-paying employer. A basic income would be an antidote to exploitative, 'flexible', zero hours 'bullshit jobs'; it would be 'the first benefit in history whose success measure is that it shrinks to zero' (Mason, 2015: 286).

There is no reason, other than exploitation, why the latest techniques of automation cannot be applied ubiquitously. We await a third managerial revolution, in the wake of which managers, trade unions and industrial system designers set their sights on networked, modular, non-linear team work. Work 'interspersed with play' could become less alienating. Networks also *disrupt*, which can be positive. 'We need to be unashamed utopians' (as were the pioneer capitalists). Significantly, Mason (2015: 288) asks: 'what is the end state?'; his response: 'that is the wrong question'. Summoning Bhasker, we inhabit an open system, and detailed blueprints constrain and call to mind ideologies with more than a hint of totalitarianism. 'So instead of looking for an end state, it's more important to ask how we might deal with reverses – or escape a dead end' (Mason, 2015: 289).

It is easy to succumb to the numbness and passivity of TINA; yet surely 'it is absurd that we are capable of witnessing a 40,000-year-old system of gender oppression begin to dissolve before our eyes and yet still see the abolition of a 200-year-old economic system as an unrealist utopia' (Mason, 2015: 290). If, as Streeck contends, financial capitalism is imploding, fracturing the societies it permeates and colonises, then alternatives of the kind Mason hints at surely wait in the wings? 'The 99% are coming to the rescue. Postcapitalism will set you free' (Mason, 2015: 292).

I have lingered awhile on Mason's diagnosis, prognosis and aspirations for a number of reasons. It is not because I am willing to underwite or sign up to his programme of reforms in its entirely (and I recognise also the limitations of my scholarship). But I do: (a) admire him for delving into 'absences' that others overlook; (b) think it a vital and pressing requirement that sociologists follow his lead; (c) applaud his focus on capitalism, warts and all; and (d) share his and Urry's conviction that alternate futures in general are important, critical and urgent objects of study for transformatory – and emancipatory – change.

If the arguments of previous chapters are on the right lines, it follows that the maldistribution of health and longevity is in significant part a function of the strategic decision-making of the capital monopolists, supported by the capital auxiliaries and 'sleepers' together with kindred spirits from lower class strata. It is then as apt as it is rare that examining sustainable alternative futures *that also open the door to a meaningful reduction in health inequalities* should pursue Streeck via the likes of Mason into a post-neoliberal economics of postcapitalism. This has been hinted elsewhere under the rubric of *permanent reform* (Scambler & Scambler, 2015). Permanent reform acknowledges the need for a revolutionary transition to postcapitalism and commends collective action to achieve a linked bundle of reforms that – together – bring a legitimation crisis closer. The kind of legitimation crisis that Habermas (1975) analysed on the cusp of financial capitalism still seems the most promising avenue for structural change.

As many analysts and commentators have recorded, the dedicated meta-reflexives and kindred spirits more readily achieve consensus on the present they oppose, with all its increasingly conspicuous power 2 relations and constraining ills, than on an absent future to which it might, with purposeful collective intent, a trigger or two and a goodly helping of serendipity and luck, succumb. Many a past utopian blueprint, I have implied, has been a carrier for some form of totalitarianism. But this is not so of Giddens's (1990) 'utopian realism', or indeed of Urry's alternative futures. And perhaps my own view has shifted a bit: I accept the need for *strong 'narratives for the future', for transformatory or emancipatory change, that bind together those multiple and largely autonomous initiatives that might, and if they are to precipitate a legitimation crisis en route to a postcapitalist and post-fractured society, 'must', mesh into a strategy of permanent reform.* In today's postindustrial world, there is no revolutionary proletariat waiting in the wings.

As Honneth (2017) argues, in the absence of an imminent working class 'for-itself', the socialist project must work at a (Mason-like) experimental piloting of alternative narratives and policies.

Winlow et al. (2016) make a significant and relevant point here. Whatever the merits of rights- and identity-based campaigns, some of which have been very effective, the transition they typically mark is a departure: (a) *from* an emphasis on a community-based culture emanating from grand narratives of 'the good society' (b) *to* an emphasis on an individualised culture privileging 'difference' (often wrongly equated with cultural tolerance) emanating from the pick-and-mix petit narratives of a relativised or postmodern culture. The effect of this cultural turn is stark and presents a very real obstacle both to the formation of compelling narratives for change towards better societal forms, and to those kinds of collective action required to pursue them.

8 A sociological Manifesto

One premise for a sociology for the twenty-first century has been implicit throughout this text. There can be no half-way decent sociology of health inequalities that is not also a sociology both of the economics of capitalism and of past, present and future societies. It must also be active rather than passive. Winlow et al. (2017: 55) are characteristically blunt:

> as one moves up the governmental, academic and media systems, the class-hierarchy becomes clear – almost all total liberal middle-class dominance. There is room for some working-class individuals, but only if they conform, and more often than not they are restricted to the lower echelons of the hierarchy. In academia's Social Science and Humanities disciplines, the most important for political education, a hierarchy dominated by the ideologies of right-wing and left-wing liberalism is reproduced by league tables, gross inequalities in research income and the maintenance of prestige among a snobbish population keen on introducing their children to the right social networks. The liberal mass media assist by promoting the work of established liberal intellectuals to the status of global stars, despite the predictability and mediocrity of their work. Liberals will fully accept individuals in the higher echelons of the hierarchy only when they become fully like them in the display of cultural and symbolic capital – people from the former working class now know this, and many pre-emptively adopt the symbols of conformity as early as possible.

Sadly, this paragraph has much applicability to sociology in general and to the sociology of health inequalities in particular: 'looking the other way' and 'asking other questions' are expedient but cowardly forms of passivity and, to my mind, constitute an abandonment of the classic sociological project.

In a paper 20 years ago I outlined and defended sociology's project as I saw it (Scambler, 1996). I drew on Habermas's critical theory sketched earlier and have not significantly changed my views since, though I would now temper them by addressing the absence of an ontology in Habermas's writings. Like Habermas, I was then and am now unconvinced by claims that we have entered an era of 'postmodernity'; indeed, I have in my own work preferred the term 'high modernity' to the more prejudicial 'late modernity' (Scambler and Higgs, 1999). Streeck may be correct in his view that capitalism is imploding, and my interpretation of British society as fractured plausible, but, as so often, babies should be rescued before they reach the plug: modernity and capitalism are not synonyms.

Kant characterised the European Enlightenment – the epitome of modernity – as a self-conscious movement indicating a human (albeit a white, male, bourgeois) progression towards 'maturity'. He promoted a concept of reason that held the promise of the fuller comprehension and control of nature and of the good society. It was a view that elicited two principal critiques. First, it seemed clear that the Enlightenment promise, more than two centuries later, had not been delivered, most notably concerning the rational construction of the good society. And second, philosophical flaws were noted in Kant's notion of reason. Both critiques have merit of course. What Habermas (1981: 9) contended, however, was that the 'project of modernity' was 'incomplete' and that it would be a mistake to abandon it:

> the project of modernity, formulated in the eighteenth century by the philosophers of the Enlightenment, consisted in their efforts to develop objective science, universal morality and law, and autonomous art according to their inner logic. At the same time, this project intended to release the cognitive potentials of each of these domains from their esoteric forms. The Enlightenment philosophers wanted to utilise this accumulation of specialised culture for the enrichment of everyday life – that is to say, for the rational organisation of everyday life.

In many ways, the entire corpus of Habermas can be interpreted as a steadfast defence of a *reconstructed* version of this project (most insistently against counter-Enlightenment thinkers like Nietzsche, Heidegger and Bataille).

Habermas rejected a Weberian commitment to irretrievably distinct 'value spheres' (i.e. science, morality/law and art), preferring instead to stress the universality of reason. Reason, he maintained, no longer has its roots in the subject-object relations of the philosophy of consciousness – 'be it the "transcendental", unhistorical subject of Kant's "pure reason" or the global subject behind Hegel's picture of Reason's "externalization" and reabsorption in history, or the privileged historical subject (the working class) of Marxist thought' (Brand, 1990: 10) – but in the subject–subject relations of communicative action. Communicative action, it will be remembered, is action oriented to understanding, which is contrasted with strategic action, or action oriented to success, often via exploitation or oppression.

Habermas charges Weber with conflating the logic and the dynamic of development. In other words, Weber treated the ('iron cage') rationalisation that has in fact occurred in the Occident as inevitable when it was contingent and selective. However understandable, the prognostic gloom found in his work and that of Habermas's predecessors at Frankfurt, especially Hork-heimer and Adorno (1972), is misconceived. After the manner of Parsons and with a hint of Luhmann, Habermas accepts that the dynamic, if not the logic, of development has meant that system rationalisation (and coloni-sation) has outstripped the rationalisation of the lifeworld. In other words, communicative action, the lifeblood of the lifeworld, has been subject to tourniquet by the system's twin steering media, money (from the economic subsystem) and power (from the subsystem of the state). Habermas locates hope for future lifeworld rationalisation in the reconstitution of its public sphere via new, as opposed to old class-based, social movements; but he is appropriately cautious. There is no easy and sure-fire means for approxi-mating to the 'ideal speech situation' that is the philosophical bedrock of the mundane, everyday interaction that comprises the lifeworld.

Habermas rejects utopian prophecy in favour of 'reasoned hope'. I wrote:

> a strong case can be made for arguing that while much sociological work arising out of unreconstructed Enlightenment thinking has proved to be flawed ..., and the idea of a postmodernist sociology is internally incon-sistent, both reason and hope are to be found in a critically-oriented so-ciology at once appropriate to high modernity and allied to Habermas' reconstructed project. This commitment to the further rationalisation of the lifeworld, grounded in Habermas' theory of communicative ac-tion, is of the essence of the critical sociology commended here ...
>
> (Scambler, 1996: 572)

I went on to defend the five 'metatheoretical' theses outlined in Table 8.1. A precis of this quintet will have to suffice. The world we inhabit is constituted through reflexively applied knowledge and subject to constant revision. Sociology it-self has become reflexive (Giddens, 1990). The (unreconstructed) Enlighten-ment ideal of certain knowledge is defunct and has, and must be, abandoned. Sociology's origins betray an affinity with this outmoded Enlightenment ideal and so, unsurprisingly, its history is one of abetting as much as resisting system rationalisation (I referenced the McDonadlisation of academic life, a phenom-enon far more relevant now than in 1996). Two illustrative examples of soci-ology's 'taming' were cited: its passivity in the face of: (a) the Thatcher-Major health care reforms (favouring markets and introducing PFIs) and (b) the Thatcherite prioritising of (individualised) cultural/behavioural over (social) material/structural explanations of health inequalities.

At the core of my argument was the assertion that sociology's overriding – logical and moral – commitment is to lifeworld rationalisation. Its system ties were, and remain, disproportionately strong, too often privileging strategic action and lifeworld colonisation over communicative action and lifeworld ra-tionalisation (Habermas, 1984, 1987; Scambler, 1987). Sociology's commitment to lifeworld rationalisation demands the pursuit of substantive (as opposed to formal, parliamentary) democracy. Substantive democracy entails further

Table 8.1 Theses towards a Critical Sociology

---
1 The full ramifications of the reflexivity of high modernity for sociological practice have been insufficiently addressed;
2 Sociology needs to more critically examine its primary allegiance to economy and state and, via the media of money and power, system rationalisation;
3 Sociology's principal commitment is to the rationalisation of the lifeworld;
4 The nature of sociology's commitment to lifeworld rationalisation requires its promotion of and engagement in a reconstituted public sphere;
5 If sociology is to be effective in promoting and engaging in a reconstituted public sphere, alliances must arguably be built with system-based and, especially, lifeworld-based activists.

Source: Adapted from Scambler (1996).

rationalisation of the lifeworld via the reconstitution of the public sphere out of the residue of a bourgeois public sphere, once progressive and resistant to economy and state but long since 'collapsed into a sham world of image creation and opinion management in which the diffusion of media products is in the service of vested interests' (Thompson, 1995: 177). This is not of course a task for sociologists alone. 'Movement intellectuals' of one kind or another might ally with the cause; and in relation to health issues:

> ... it seems clear first that the state cannot move to neutralise many current threats to the people's health through political or structural change without contradiction and without risking a crisis, ultimately of legitimation ...; second that many health threats can be understood as latent functions of selective – or excessive – system rationalisation in the west; third that the optimum, if presently slender, prospect for countering many health threats may rest with public mobilisation around political and structural change, contingent upon advances in substantive democracy in the public sphere of the lifeworld attained through the new politics of the new social movements; and fourth that, given overlapping (new public health) agendas, real opportunities exist for alliances between activists across the boundaries between system and lifeworld.
>
> (Scambler and Goraya, 1994: 9)

Reason, I argued, conceived formally or procedurally as universal,

> commits sociology to what Habermas has referred to as the reconstructed and as yet incomplete project of modernity; that this commitment requires that sociology be directed first and foremost to the decolonisation and further rationalisation of the lifeworld; and that this, in turn, necessitates sociologists, *fated to be actors in high modernity*, acting *consciously* through alliances of interests with other system-based and lifeworld-based activists ... to promote and engage with a reconstituted public sphere of the lifeworld.
>
> (Scambler, 1996: 579)

I was careful not to claim that all system-driven sociology is without return, nor that all sociological work defined in the context of my paper as pre- or non-critical is without value. I insisted too that, if sociology is committed to contributing to the project of modernity, there is no occasion either for utopian prophecy or even for optimism. I ended with a revealing quotation from Habermas's interview with Haller (1994: 112–113):

> the 'emancipated society' is an ideal construction that invites misunderstanding. I'd rather speak of the idea of the undisabled subject. In general, this idea can be derived from the analysis of the necessary conditions for reaching understanding – it describes something like the image of symmetric relations of the freely reciprocal recognition of communicatively interacting subjects. Of course this idea can't be depicted as the totality of a reconciled form of life and cast into the future as a utopia. It contains nothing more, but nothing less, than the formal characterisation of necessary conditions for nonanticipatable forms of an undisabled life.

As was indicated in Chapter 2, this argument has since been developed. Burawoy's (2005) delineation of four sociologies en route to his promulgation of one of them, public sociology, is widely known. Sasha Scambler and I (2015) have made a case for adding a further two. To recap, Burawoy's four sociologies comprise: (a) *professional sociology*, represented by the *scholar*; (b) *policy sociology*, represented by the *reformer*; (c) *critical sociology*, represented by the *radical*; and, his innovation, (d) *public sociology*, represented by the *democrat*. Our contribution has been to append: (e) *foresight sociology*, represented by the *visionary*; and (f) *action sociology*, represented by the *activist*. The foresight sociologist is committed, in line with Urry's exhortations, to exploring organizational-cum-institutional *alternative futures*. What kind of evidence-based options and interventions might serve to reduce health inequalities? The action sociologist cannot accept ideological dismissal resulting from power 2 relations (e.g. the governing oligarchy paying lip-service to Marmot-style recommendations while either undermining or 'kicking them into the long grass'). Action sociology, then, opposes, debunks and contests the myths that fuel distorted or pathological views of the world.

Table 8.2 complements the discussion so far with a third column specifying a thrust, mode of reasoning or 'logic' for each of the six sociologies. Logic here is intended in a sociological/informal rather than a philosophical/formal sense. Professional sociology is articulated via a *cumulative* logic; that is, it is premised on an enhanced understanding or grasp of social structures, cultures and institutions over time. Policy sociology reflects a *utilitarian* logic in that its teleological rationale is reasoned institutional reform towards the betterment of human quality of life and wellbeing. Critical sociology's logic is *meta-theoretical*. In other words, its purpose is to encourage or prompt reflexivity and accountability in its sibling sociologies. Public sociology most clearly expresses the Habermasian logic of *communicative*

Table 8.2 Six Sociologies and their Representatives and Logics

Sociologies	Sociologists	Mode of engagement
Professional	Scholar	Cumulative
Policy	Reformer	Utilitarian
Critical	Radical	Meta-theoretical
Public	Democrat	Communicative
Foresight	Visionary	Speculative
Action	Activist	Strategic

Source: Adapted from Scambler and Scambler (2015).

action (oriented to understanding and rational consensus). Foresight sociology is associated with what might be called a *speculative* mode of reasoning: it is by definition released from the time-bound constraints of the present to anticipate possible futures. Finally, action sociology gives rise to a logic of *strategic* action. Its rationale is in an important sense political, so its impulse is oriented to outcome, to be 'effective', for example to counter *and defeat* ideological misrepresentation.

In Habermasian terms, action sociology's strategic thrust creates a tension with its professional parentage; *but it is a move that in my view must be made.* Two important qualifications are in order: first, it is the *community of sociologists, not each individual*, that is obligated to deliver on action sociology; and second, in relation to this particular text, it does not follow from my privileging of class relations for explaining health inequalities within and between nation states that class invariably trumps other structures or relations – gender, ethnic and so on – across all figurations, which would be manifestly false.

I have tried to make a case for going beyond BCR to accommodate DCR in pursuit of an optimal sociological theorizing of health inequalities. DCR has the potential: (a) to reframe sociological explanation in this context, (b) to reinvigorate a sociological project buttressed by a reconstructed neo-Enlightenment philosophy and (c) to refocus our collective attention on absence, that ocean of non-being from which the tiny islet of being so easily distracts us. In Chapter 2 and above, I have sketched an agenda for a future sociology of health inequalities that owes itself to and feeds off the typology of six sociologies/sociologists/logics. In this concluding discussion, I suggest ways in which this might be translated into a research programme. But first some preliminaries.

Professional sociology

Professional sociology richly encompasses many schools of theory, perspectives, orientations and methodologies (see Chapter 2). Given the focus of this book, some general criticisms, immanent critiques, need restating or clarifying. I despair, for example, of wholly positivistic/empiricist studies whose authors nurse aspirations that are doomed from the outset. Cross-sectional and even longitudinal investigations of aggregates of individuals that target distributions of health and longevity can only describe patterns. Sociology, to my mind, unlike epidemiology, which is properly oriented to prediction in the service of public health policy and intervention, should be geared first and foremost to causal explanations. Furthermore, positivistic enquiries typically: (a) pretend to a Humean atheoretical neutrality as to what 'is'; (b) ignore or side-step commitments to what 'ought to be' (e.g. healthy or fit bodies and equitable health care); (c) operate on the false prospectus that they can, in interdisciplinary 'cumulative' combination, *wrap phenomena up*; and (d) reinforce the political status quo by sticking with – accept being bounded by – the present and ignoring absent alternative possibilities.

Consider the two statements from one of the most respected researchers of what she refers to as *health inequality* rather than health inequalities, Mel Bartley. First, she maintains that 'there are several characteristics of explanations for health inequality that could serve as a very basic set of requirements for an adequate explanation:

- explanations should be biologically plausible;
- they should show a 'dose-response relationship';
- they should extend to health differences between men and women;
- they should extend to health differences between ethnic groups;
- they should be consistent with trends for the whole population over time;
- they should be consistent with international differences (Bartley, 2017: 199).

This might seem an uncontroversial list, for all that it implies an unlikely measure of stability by social structure and culture as well as time and place. The subtext, however, is: (a) that it is only positivistic research in the guise of (lifecourse-oriented) multivariate analyses that has the potential to deliver on this 'basic set of requirements' and (b) that this whole edifice rests on Hume's notion of causality as constant conjunction complemented by Mill's canons of scientific enquiry. Krieger (2017) pointedly asks: 'can the causes of population health be parsed into components that add up to 100%'. She rightly answers no, but it sometimes seems that this is precisely positivists' aspiration.

Bhaskar notes that many non-critical realist and positivistic researchers (unreflexively) deploy retroductive inference to arrive at 'causal explanations', and Bartley does this too, but an underlying commitment to positivism, because it lacks an ontology that allows for the discernment and theorising of 'real' generative mechanisms and their powers and tendencies, retards or impairs the sociological project.

Bartley's second statement anticipates the brief of a policy sociology. She (2017: 201) writes:

as someone who occasionally gets asked questions by people who are engaged in policy debate, I would like to be able to answer, with a lot more confidence, from research that is growing organically in a connected way. Because I really don't think that it is possible to point to clear policy implications from the present state of health inequality research. What is needed is a research programme adequate to the purpose of a greater understanding of social factors in health and disease in populations. From this the policy implications will flow.

So nearly four decades after the publication of the Black Report, replete with its detailed policy recommendations and costings, it seems that we are no closer to designing and implementing effective policies to reduce health inequalities. It would take a pathologically naive inductivist – which, let's be clear, Bartley is not – to infer that another 40 years might do the trick.

Policy sociology

Policy sociology's contribution to the sociological project is an important one. To critique positivistic inputs is not to undermine, let alone dismiss it. There are two points to emphasise here. The first is that policy sociology that is truly aligned with the sociological project as defined above cannot afford to be circumscribed and tamed in line with what neoliberal universities and funding bodies are willing to sign off and subsidise. Academic sociologists now typically face role strain, discomfort and downright bullying if they opt to fight for 'untamed' careers that they cannot self-finance, with a little left over in gratitude to their line managers. Times are tougher than they were for baby boomers like me. The second point is that, if it is to be effective, policy sociology must reflexively adopt the strategy of permanent reform alluded to earlier. Only a focused orientation to reform-upon-reform towards a revolutionary transition to a post-capitalist society can do the trick. In other words, policy sociologists must become reconciled to the kind of 'evidence base' they purport to celebrate, that is, one that, for example, not only exhorts citizens-cum-consumers to cease smoking, avoid daily visits to pubs, desist from frequenting fast food outlets and eschew an overly sedentary lifestyle, *but one that pays more than lip service to challenging the increasingly transnational and pathogenic for-profit corporations that foster precisely these risk behaviours.* To 'go public', to commit to Burawoy's public sociology, is not enough.

Critical sociology

There is a sense in which this whole book can be regarded as professional-cum-critical sociology. It draws and comments on each of its companion sociologies, but it is critical sociology that it most represents and to which it mostly contributes. An exercise in critical discourse analysis offered by Bhaskar (2016: 106–109) provides a further illustration. He draws on and dissects a proto-sociological article by Hutton in *The Observer* on 29 June 2013, which provides a commentary on a financial statement by (now ex-) UK

Chancellor of the Exchequer George Osborne. First, Hutton gives a precis of the speech. Second, he offers an interpretation of the text in terms of 'political positioning', that is, 'in the context of the discursive processes of the production and intended effect of the text'. The text is thereby exposed as a 'party political stratagem'. And third, these discursive processes are related back to the state of the British economy and society, that is, 'to the social context that generates them and in which they are intended to play a role'. Hutton ends by querying the likely effectiveness of Osborne's stratagem.

Bhaskar (2016: 109) cites Fairclough (2003) but 'elaborates' when he analyses Hutton's article as a form of critical discourse analysis. Five stages are apparent:

- Focus on a social problem that has a semiotic aspect: for Bhaskar, this corresponds to an explanatory critique of a false belief or social ill, the point being to inform emancipatory change;
- Identify obstacles to its being tackled through an analysis of the network of practices in which it is located, of the relationship of semiosis to other elements within the relevant practices and of the discourse (or semiosis) itself;
- Consider whether the 'network of practices' *needs* the problem, and if so, why, plus ask what mechanisms, however circuitously, produce and reproduce it;
- Identify possible ways past the obstacles, focusing on 'hitherto unrealised possibilities for change in the way life is currently organised', thereby raising issues of 'concrete utopianism, a theory of transition and a relationship to an on-going depth struggle';
- Grasp these 'unrealised possibilities' as the object of an emancipatory practice oriented to 'the definitive resolution of the social problem or ill'.

Bhaskar's interpretation of Fairclough adds flesh to the bones of a critical sociology.

Public sociology

Burawoy's advocacy of public sociology points to a sociological engagement with the enabling and protest sectors of civil society that meaningfully permeates the public sphere and travels well beyond publication in peer-review journals. After all, who but career academics read such formal and arcane pieces? In the context of the present inspection of health inequalities, perhaps the best model for public British sociology, irony of ironies, is Wilkinson and Pickett's (2009) *epidemiological* excursion via their *The Spirit Level*. In this path-breaking book, its authors argued, *accessibly* as well as persuasively, that the more unequal a (putatively 'developed') society, the more social problems – from criminal, extending to homicidal and suicidal propensities, to the marginally more mundane matter of health disparities – significantly accrue and impact. Their statistics have been disputed, as is to be expected; *but* an element of this disputation has undoubtedly been ideological. There is a painful lesson for sociologists here. It is one thing to traverse civil society's enabling sector en route to its protest sector in a public sphere Habermas judged 'refeudalised', and quite another to prosper, let alone survive, there. To proclaim as much is to anticipate a tension central to action sociology (see below).

Foresight sociology

Excepting the contributions of innovative practitioners like Urry, there has been a tendency for sociologists to: (a) neglect alternative futures and, (b) when they have engaged, to anticipate 'catastrophic' dystopias rather than inspiring and realisable concrete utopias. The objection that to trade in concrete utopias is to turn sociology from a scientific to a normative exercise is premised on the Humean dichotomy between 'is' and 'ought' that was queried earlier. Few see difficulties in engaging in scientific research *because we ought to* tackle diseases; perhaps more baulk at engaging in scientific research *because we ought to* tackle health inequalities. In both examples, however, the scientific project reveals an explicit moral thrust. According to the characterisation of the (reconstructed) Enlightenment project of sociology I have advanced in this volume, this normativity is logically inscribed in professional sociology and assumes the form of lifeworld rationalisation. We need more Mason-like exegeses. Anticipating the next section on action sociology, there is an obvious affinity between this commitment to lifeworld rationalisation and Bhaskar's transformation model.

Action sociology

Professional sociology has, in my view been, overly casual in responding to, taking on board and ceding intellectual territory to a diverse and fruitful array of understandably and rightfully rebellious consociates, including feminist, ethnic/post-colonial and disability studies (see Chapter 2). As professional sociologists, we should in my view listen to, reflect on and embrace (but obviously *not* attempt to territorialise or colonise) these domains. I appreciate that it will be hard to earn trust. Sociology in the absence of these emancipatory forces has indubitably become more bourgeois, respectable and tamed. Professional sociology's investigations of gender, ethnicity and disability are still all too often masculine, white, ableist and anodyne. But this is to anticipate the agendas of critical, public, foresight and action sociologies.

Two further comments are significant here. If, first, I am right to argue that a sociological project for the twenty-first century is logically and morally focused on lifeworld rationalisation, then this sits comfortably with – has what might be called an elective affinity with – Bhaskar's critical realist approach to transformation and emancipation. His transformational model was introduced earlier (see Chapters 3 and 5). I pick up here on his DCR account of transformative praxis (specifically, '4D', that is, his zone of transformative agency), which meshes with his ethics. The most telling absence that DCR overcomes is the absence of absence, or negativity, change, which allows 'a kind of recursive definition of dialectic as absenting absences of constraints on absenting ills ... to further human progress we need to absent ill, or ill being' (Bhaskar, 2017: 88–89). Bhaskar's concept of explanatory critique is, in the proverbial nutshell, *for* improving wellbeing and *against* the ills that stand in, clutter and obstruct its various paths. Starting from the simple notion of agentive freedom, Bhaskar systematically broaches more complex notions like that of emancipation, autonomy, wellbeing and flourishing.

Bhaskar adumbrates seven forms of freedom, which are summarised in Table 8.3. It begins with a straightforward concept of agential freedom and of 'negative and positive freedoms' and moves through progressively more complex concepts of emancipation, autonomy, wellbeing and flourishing. Finally, 'at the end of the ethical dialectic is a society in which we are oriented to the free flourishing of each, as a condition of the free flourishing of all' (Bhaskar, 2017: 90). Bhaskar acknowledges an indebtedness to Marx's concept of a communist society, now being 'recovered' in the writings of left theorists like Badiou, when he writes of eudaimonia, for a eudaimonistic society is oriented to human wellbeing or flourishing. Bhaskar (2017: 91–92) again:

> The eudaimonistic society, the goal put forward by dialectical critical realism, depends on the transcendence of all master/slave-type relations. Here it is useful to distinguish between two concepts of power: power 1, which is transformative capacity, and power 2, which is oppression. Clearly what we need to do is for the oppressed to have more of power 1 in order to transform the power 2 relation between their oppressors and themselves and in order to transform the relationship itself ... The other thing perhaps to mention is in the ethical dialectic of dialectical critical realism; a big role is played by what I call the logic of dialectical universalised ability. We can get the gist of this logic by looking at two kinds of ethical dialectics that it postulates. The first, the dialectic of desire or agency: this proceeds from an agent having a desire. Then what is argued is that this desire contains with it a meta-desire to abolish any constraints on that desire. The logic of universalised ability insists that an agent so committed must logically be committed to the abolition of all dialectically similar constraints. And so it moves in the direction and necessitates a solidarity with others. Similarly, in the dialectic of discourse the starting point is the expressive veracity of statements of

Table 8.3 Forms of Freedom

1 **Agentive freedom:** the power to start/act anew;
2 **Negative or positive freedom:** be free from constraints on/to be free to do;
3 **Emancipation:** universal human emancipation from (unnecessary) constraints;
4 **Autonomy:** possess the power, knowledge and disposition to act in real interests;
5 **Wellbeing:** the absence of ills;
6 **Flourishing:** the realisation of possibilities;
7 **Eudaimonia:** universal human flourishing.

Source: From Bhaskar (2017).

solidarity, which entail commitment to the person and situation one is in solidarity with, entailing action, which again, proceeding through the logic of universalised ability, will be aimed at the transformation of all dialectically similar constraints, and ultimately all dialectical constraints of human freedom and flourishing as such.

I have quoted Bhaskar at length here both as a reminder of the summary discussion of dialectical critical realism in Chapter 5 and, beyond that, to suggest that, rescued from its narrow and 'privileged' origins in the late-eighteenth century European Enlightenment, the sociological project is allied to Bhaskar's seventh form of freedom. If not, what is sociology *for*?

My second comment is more prosaic and perhaps more awkward to satisfy. Public sociology, it was claimed, deploys a logic of communicative action, that is, one oriented to consensual understanding. Action sociology, on the other hand, is characterised by a logic of strategic action, namely, one oriented to outcome. Marx, and Machiavelli most notably before him, recognised that accomplishing change requires more than a commitment to Burawoy's four sociologies. Power 2 relations, epitomised in the class/command dynamic and propagandised via a family of neoliberal repertoires, are not susceptible to reason and evidence alone. If they were, the NHS would not now be in the process of being sold off. Wilkinson and Pickett pursued a form of public epidemiology (via their *The Spirit Level*), only to be assaulted by unreason and non-evidence. They have continued to present and represent reason and evidence on a website and on social media; but to what effect? And this is the nub of my concern. If in action sociology the logic of communicative action is displaced by that of strategic action, there are surely net cons as well as pros. It is one thing to commend or champion emancipatory transformative change, quite another to bring it about. My preference for coalitions around a general platform of permanent reform presumes *effectiveness*; indeed, without it, it retreats into an anodyne and benign kind of public sociology, or professional sociology writ just a tad larger.

For all that I judge the sociological project to be logically and morally committed to lifeworld rationalisation, which implies a willingness to contest ideological opposition *and more*, I have yet to come fully to terms with my own version of action sociology. Consider the 'gap' between Marx's triad on *Capital* and *The Communist Manifesto* he penned with Engels, the former a (non-bourgeois, proto-sociological) analysis, the latter a translation of analysis into an all-out call to arms. In his and Engels's lives, the analysis and the call to arms were fused. What I can and do advocate here is an engagement on the part of the sociological community *as a whole* 'for' evidence based policy and 'against' policy based evidence. And this amounts, for example, to combatting policies designed to grant impunity to transnational corporations peddling health risks as commodities and to make accessible the 'NHS brand' to for-profit interlopers. If there continues to be an imbalance across the six sociologies – for example, too few sociologists commit too little to foresight and action sociology – then there is a sense in which even professional sociology, sitting at the very core of the discipline and characterised by scholarship and cumulative understanding and explanation, elides, as it were by default, into a kind of non-action sociology that conforms more to a strategic than to a cumulative, utilitarian, meta-theoretical or communicative logic. In other words, *not* engaging in action sociology becomes a dominant form of non-decision-making that amounts to a 'camouflaged' form of decision-making.

I end with a provisional series of macro-, meso- and micro-oriented queries about our fractured society and its health inequalities that to my mind prefigure a fit-for-purpose research programme for the twenty-first century. These are outlined in Table 8.4. Unsurprisingly given the preceding discussion, the focus is on society's fracturing rather than the socio-epidemiological studies, often misrepresented as quantitative sociology, that continue to dominate the field.

The rationale for the presentation of this series of queries should by now be apparent, so I will not labour the point by dwelling on it further, but rather draw the study to a conclusion by restating the convictions upon which it has been based. There are few (if any) sociologists who would deny the role of social structures in producing, reproducing and deepening health inequalities, for all that they often differ in defining and, perhaps more to the point, operationalising them. For many, a neo-positivist measurement, via the transmutation of social phenomena into statistics-friendly variables, is a vital ingredient for doing social *science*. I demur: I insist, for example, that the tricky problem of operationalising ever-changing asset flows pertinent to health and longevity fades away once a critical realist perspective displaces a neo-positivist one. To repeat, this is neither to dismiss the notion that there are sociological lessons to be learned from neo-positivist research, nor to critique socio-epidemiological research oriented to public health. But it is to reassert the primacy for all forms of science of the 'real' and of retroductive and abductive searches for those generative mechanisms – at macro-, meso- and micro-levels – most salient for health and life expectancy. While it seems implicit in much neo-positivistic research that it will one day be possible to 'wrap up' a sociology of health inequalities, I prefer the more modest sociological aspiration to 'make a case' in a dynamic and shifting, not to mention fractured, social landscape.

Table 8.4 Future Research Programme for a Sociology of Health Inequalities

	Macro-sociological questions	Meso-sociological questions	Micro-sociological questions
Professional sociology	Are capitalism's days numbered? Is the class/command dynamic *the* crucial morphogenetic cycle in financial capitalism? How do 'systemic' social structures contribute to susceptibility to disease and premature mortality? What is the relative causal salience of structures like class, gender, ethnicity and age in figurations like the nation state and the global arena? To what extent are cultural shifts pertinent for health and longevity down to structural change? Which theories of contemporary society and social change cast most light on these structural issues? To what extent are class alignments and 'consciousness' compromised by cultural changes? Is a 'legitimation crisis' imminent, and is it the most likely precipitant of structural change?	To what extent do the asset flows, effort-reward imbalance, risk aversion, ego adjustment and activity reinforcement models constitute mechanisms that translate macro- into micro-forces for health inequalities? How might those heterogeneous and complex class and command relations most salient for health inequalities be optimally 'unpacked' figuration-by-figuration? How salient is neoliberal ideology for enacting structures that deepen health inequalities? To what extent have 'grand' narratives for identity and change been translated into relativised 'petit' narratives, and with what consequences for health inequalities? How are Mills's 'tacit understanding' and 'high morality' sustained?	Which 'artful', mundane or everyday interactions serve (a) to reproduce, or (b) to transform those meso- and macro-mechanisms that are pivotal for health inequalities? How, in the lifeworld, do strategic class and command decisions intrude and shape thinking and behaviour? How is the present 'sociology of health inequalities' underpinned and presented 'as is'? Just how, day-to-day, do the unintended consequences of sociologists' behaviours deliver 'against' their intent? If everyday interaction is mediated by socially induced reflexivity, what are the thresholds for negotiation?

Policy sociology	Which policies promise an effective return on the reduction of health inequalities? To what extent are these effective policies compromised by coalitions of wealth and power? How are society-wide relations of gender, ethnicity and age subverted by policy discourse and rhetoric? How and to what/whose ends is stigma 'weaponised'?	How might the tension between effective policy formation and implementation and the forces resisting them be optimally managed? How, and to what degree, does the post-1970s neoliberalisation of universities tame researchers? Does research funding ultimately determine findings and applicability? What are the mechanisms that translate stigma into deviance? In accordance with which mechanisms does evidence-based policy translate into policy-based evidence? Does the concept of 'evidence-based medicine' have any lingering relevance to tackling health inequalities?	In accordance with which day-to-day dynamics might effective policy-making be compromised? How is the taming of researchers practically accomplished? What follows from another grant, another high-impact article? How do sociologists collaborate their way towards the status of 'collaborationists'? How are shame and blame acted out in the lifeworld? How salient are felt stigma and deviance for definitions of self?
Critical sociology	How might the respectability of the sociology of health inequalities best be interrogated?	What are the mechanisms according to which sociology's respectability is anchored institutionally?	How does everyday decision-making in sociology structure (if not structurally determine) the reproduction versus the transformation of the status quo?
Public sociology	How, and in line with which structures or relations, does the dissemination of sociological theory and research impact on political and practice? What comprises the public sphere in the twenty-first century?	How do different media – mainstream versus social – encapsulate or contest sociological interests? To what extent do institutional incentives to 'public engagement' satisfy/frustrate public sociology?	How is 'going public' accomplished? Do mundane decisions and actions constrain/enable career choices? How does agency and reflexivity contribute to what sociology is and becomes?

(Continued)

	Macro-sociological questions	Meso-sociological questions	Micro-sociological questions
Foresight sociology	How does what 'might be' compare with what 'is' in the sociological canon? How does sociology – intrinsically versus extrinsically – relate to visionary change? What evidence favours 'this' rather than 'that' option for reducing health inequalities exists?	Are there compelling scenarios for experiments for effective change? Are there natural and thought-experiments 'out there' to be investigated? Does foresight sociology herald career advantages/disadvantages?	In what contexts do sociologists 'choose' to 'do' alternative futures? How key is institutional self-presentation, via public engagement, for foresight sociology?
Action sociology	When and how does sociology become (irredeemably) 'bourgeois'? When does 'sticking with' communicative action amount to a strategic choice? What are the 'de jure' and 'de facto' prerequisites for a sociology committed to the good society and to human flourishing?	How do 'insider' versus 'outsider' routes to change compare? By which routes do institutional line-managers turn into proponents of the status quo? What is the role of funding agencies, and to what extent, and how, do they lean to the status quo? Are there mechanisms that facilitate the rationalisation of 'quietude'?	How do day-to-day options translate into 'political' commitments? To what extent, and how, do 'internal conversations' reflect macro- and meso-mechanisms? How do sociologists 'do' reflexivity? By what means does reflexivity deliver passivity?
Most salient perspectives/ Schools of thought	Stuctural-functionalism; post-structuralism and postmodernism; social constructionism; conflict and critical theory; feminist and post-colonial theory; critical realism.	Structural-functionalism; post-structuralism and postmodernism; conflict and critical theory; feminist and post-colonial theory; critical realism.	Interactionism; phenomenology and ethnomethodology; feminist and post-colonial theory; critical realism.

Another related theme running throughout is a critique of: (a) a lack of sociological ambition in health inequalities research (Marx would understandably have dismissed much of it as bourgeois pseudo-science) and (b) the supine attitude of the sociological community in the face of attempts to block its findings via the systemic colonisation – that is, class-sponsored and command-policed penetration – of civil society and the public sphere of the lifeworld. Allied to this is the promotion of action and foresight sociologies informed by a dialectical notion of absence (negating negation and the absenting of constraining ills rooted in power 2 relations), that is, setting off not from what is present but from what is not and what might be. This is to my mind what affords purpose and leverage to sociology as part of a reconstructed Enlightenment project. If Bhaskar delivers an ontology, Habermas contributes too by means of his theory of communicative action. It should go without saying that there are lessons to be learned from the only-too-positive splinterings of the likes of feminist, post-colonial and disability activist theories and studies from distracted and wayward sociological parenting.

Coming to the end of a book sharpens awareness of its limitations. It has been argued, in effect, that the macro-social class/command relations of financial capitalism that have given birth by caesarean section to a fractured society might be seen as one of Archer's morphogenic cycles and one, moreover, which is of paramount importance for a sociology of health inequalities. Some elaboration of this has been posited via the specification of meso-social mechanisms consonant with empirical findings. Less attention has been paid to micro-social interaction, though Table 8.4 logs pressing questions.

The focus on the class/command dynamic has nudged aside many another social structure. This has been justified as a corrective to the sustained neglect of social class as a core generative mechanism in the figuration of the nation state, rather than as a proxy variable that absents the capitalist executive. Obviously, this does not imply that other structures/mechanisms are unimportant. To recall the jigsaw model, the logics of patriarchy and tribalism that issue in structures or relations of gender and ethnicity respectively can and do rival and trump class in many figurations (but rarely, I suggest, in that of the contemporary, Occidental nation state). There exist excellent discussions of gender and ethnicity and health and health inequalities elsewhere, most recently under the generic rubric of intersectionalism. In short, I have here merely fitted in a few (I would say key, even helpful) pieces of a complex 5000 word+ jigsaw.

It needs emphasizing that the twenty-first century *sociological project*, part and parcel of a Habermasian reconstructed project of modernity – namely, one geared to social transformation towards a 'good society' that allows for 'human flourishing', even if this involves enigmatic (Kant and Hegel via Marx to Bhaskar) assertions that we must absent absence – is what I think sociology is about. A strong, skillful and committed professional sociology is a basic requirement: the other five sociologies follow on. And it is the sociological community as a whole rather than its individual members who owe coverage to all six sociologies. If not, what?

Kayleigh Garthwaite (2016) conducted an ethnographic study of a Trussel Trust foodbank in Stockton-on-Tees. In the course of her discussion of hardship beyond-the-pale, she cites five sets of circumstances in which citizens have been 'sanctioned'; that is, had their benefits suspended for personal irresponsibility:

- a man was sanctioned after he missed an appointment because he took his mother to chemotherapy;
- a woman had an interview which lasted longer than she expected, so she was 10 minutes late for her job centre appointment and was sanctioned for a month;
- a man was sanctioned for being 2 minutes late, even though he had turned up 15 minutes early but wasn't allowed to go upstairs to see his adviser until the security guard said so;
- another man missed an appointment after he travelled to Scotland for a family funeral for four members of his family who had been killed in a car crash by a drunk driver. He was sanctioned, even though he rang the job centre to tell them he wouldn't be there;
- a woman who went on a health and social care course the job centre sent her on was sanctioned for not going to her job centre appointment, even though she was on the course the job centre had sent her on (Garthwaite, 2016: 84).

So a system set in place by a millionaire government minister, Ian Duncan Smith, and overseen by his department, that of Work and Pensions, administered by a for-profit firm rewarded for its rate of sanctioning, persecuted and took already desperate people's trust and hope away. Too often in financial capitalism and the divisive and fractured society it has spawned this is how the asset flows needed for health and longevity are strangled. Sanctioning seeps quietly into people's body systems. In this new Dickensian Britain, it is surely time for sociologists to follow Virchow and Engels into a political field that, as Bourdieu (1980) rightly insists, influences all other fields.

References

Acheson Report (1998) The Independent Inquiry into Inequalities in Health. London; HMSO.

Anderson, R, Hughes, J & Sturrock, W (1986) Philosophy and the Human Sciences. London; Croom Helm.

Annendale, E (2009) Women's Health and Social Change. London; Routledge.

Archer, M (1979) Social Origins of Educational Systems. London; Sage.

Archer, M (1988) Culture and Agency: The Place of Culture in Social Theory. Cambridge, UK; Cambridge University Press.

Archer, M (1995) Realist Social Theory: The Morphogenetic Approach. Cambridge, UK; Cambridge University Press.

Archer, M (2000) Being Human: The Problem of Agency. Cambridge, UK; Cambridge University Press.

Archer, M (2007a) The trajectory of the morphogenetic approach: An account in the first person. *Sociologica, Problemas e Practicas* 54 35–47.

Archer, M (2007b) The ontological status of subjectivity: The missing link between structure and agency. In Eds Lawson, C, Latsis, J & Martins, N: Contributions to Social Ontology. London; Routledge.

Archer, M (2007c) Making Our Way in the World. Cambridge, UK; Cambridge University Press.

Archer, M (2012) The Reflexive Imperative. Cambridge, UK; Cambridge University Press.

Archer, M (2013) Social morphogenesis and the project of morphogenetic society. In Ed Archer, M: Social Morphogenesis. New York; Springer.

Archer, M (2014) The generative mechanism re-configuring late modernity. In Ed Archer, M: Late Modernity: Trajectories Towards Morphogenetic Society. New York; Springer.

Armstrong, D (1987) Theoretical trends in biopsychosocial medicine. *Social Science and Medicine* 25 1213–1218.

Armstrong, D (1995) The rise of surveillance medicine. *Sociology of Health and Illness* 17 393–404.

Badiou, A (2016) Pocket Pantheon. London; Verso.

Baert, P (1998) Social Theory in the Twentieth Century. Cambridge, UK; Polity Press.

Bambra, C (2016) Health Divides: Where You Live Can Kill You. Bristol, UK; Policy Press.

Barnes, C & Mercer, G (2003) Disability. Cambridge, UK; Polity Press.

Bartley, M (2017) Health Inequality: An Introduction to Theories, Concepts and Methods, 2nd ed. Cambridge, UK; Polity Press.

Bauman, Z (1976) The Active Utopia. London; Allen Unwin.

Bauman, Z (1987) Legislators and Interpreters: On Modernity, Postmodernity and Intellectuals. Cambridge, UK; Cambridge University Press.

Bauman, Z (2000) Liquid Modernity. Cambridge, UK; Polity Press.

Bauman, Z (2007) Liquid Times: Living in an Age of Uncertainty. Cambridge, UK; Polity Press.

Bauman, Z (2011) Culture in a Liquid Modern World. Cambridge, UK; Polity Press.

Beck, U (1982) Risk Society. London; Sage.

Beresford, P (2014) Rich List 2014: The Definitive Guide to Wealth in Britain and Ireland. *Sunday Times*.

Bernstein, R (1976) The Restructuring of Social and Political Theory. London; Methuen.

Beveridge, W (1942) Social Insurance and Allied Services. Cmnd 6404. London; HMSO.

Bhambra, (2015) Connected Sociologies. London; Bloomsbury.

Bhaskar, R (1987) The Possibility of Naturalism: A Philosophical Critique of the Contemporary Human Sciences, 2nd ed. Hemel Hempstead; Harvester Wheatsheaf.

Bhaskar, R (1993) Dialectic: The Pulse of Freedom. London; Verso.

Bhaskar, R (1998) Critical realism and dialectical. In Eds Archer, M, Bhaskar, R, Collier, A, Lawson, T & Norrie, A: Critical Realism: Essential Readings. Londfon; Routledge.

Bhaskar, R (2016) Enlightened Common Sense: The Philosophy of Critical Realism. London; Routledge.

Bhasker, R (2017) The Order of Natural Necessity. London; Routledge.

Bhaskar, R, Danermark, B & Price, L (2017) Interdisciplinarity and Well-Being: A Critical Realist General Theory of Interdisciplinarity. London; Routledge.

Bhaskar, R & Norrie, A (1998) Dialectic and dialectical critical realism. In Eds Archer, M, Bhaskar, R, Collier, A, Lawson, T & Norrie, A: Critical Realism: Essential Readings. London; Routledge.

Black, D (1982) Inequalities in Health: The Black Report. London; Penguin Books.

Blumer, H (1969) Symbolic Interactionism: Perspectives and Methods. New York; Prentice-Hall.

Bourdieu, R (1980) The Logic of Practice. Cambridge, UK; Polity Press.

Braaten, J (1991) Habermas' Critical Theory of Society. New York; State University of New York Press.

Brand, A (1990) The Force of Reason: An Introduction to Habermas' 'Theory of Communicative Action'. London; Allen & Unwin.

Brock, T, Carrigan, M & Scambler, G (2017) Introduction. In Eds Brock, T, Carrigan, M & Scambler, G: Structure, Culture and Agency: Selected Papers of Margaret Archer. London; Taylor & Francis.

Brown, A (2002) Developing realistic philosophy: from critical realism to materialistic dialectics. In Eds Brown, A, Fleetwood, S & Roberts, A: Critical Realism and Marxism. London; Routledge.

Brown, G & Harris, T (1978) Social Origins of Depression. London; Tavistock.

Buechler, S (2008) Critical Sociology. Boulder, CO; Paradigm Publishers.

Burawoy, M (2005) For public sociology. *American Sociological Review* 70 4–28.

Bury, M (1986) Social constructionism and the development of medical sociology. *Sociology of Health and Illness* 8 137–169.

Bury, M (1987) Social constructionism and medical sociology: A rejoinder to Nicolson and McLaughlin. *Sociology of Health and Illness* 9 439–444.

Carroll, W (2008) The corporate elite and the transformation of financial capital. In Eds Savage, M & Williams, K: Remembering Elites. Oxford; Blackwell.

Castells, M (1996) The Rise of the Network Society. Vol.1: The Information Age: Economy, Society and Culture. Oxford; Blackwell.

Castells, M (2009) Communication Power. Oxford; Oxford University Press.

Castells, M (2010a) The Rise of the Network Society. Vol.1: The Information Age: Economy, Society and Culture, 2nd ed. Oxford; Blackwell.

Castells, M (2010b) The Information Age: Economy, Society and Culture. Volume 1: Rise of the Network Society, 2nd ed. Oxford; Blackwell.

Castells, M (2012) Networks of Outrage and Hope: Social Movements in the Internet Age. Cambridge, UK; Polity Press.

Clark, T & Heath, A (2014) Hard Times: The Divisive Toll of the Economic Slump. New Haven, CT; Yale University Press.

Chadwick, E (1842) Report on the Sanitary Condition of the Labouring Population of Great Britain.

Clement, W & Myles, J (1997) Relations of Ruling: Class and Gender in Postindustrial Societies. Toronto; McGill Queen's University Press.

Coburn, D (2009) Inequality and health. In Eds Panitch, L & Leys, C: Morbid Symptoms: Health under Capitalism. Pontypool, UK; Merlin Press.

Cockerham, W (2000) Medical sociology at the millennium. In Eds Quah, S & Sales, A: The International Handbook of Sociology. London; Sage.

Cockerham, W (2013) Sociological theory in medical sociology in the early twenty-first century. *Social Theory and Health* 11 241–255.

Collier, A (1994) Critical Realism: An Introduction to Roy Bhaskar's Philosophy. London; Verso.

Collier, A (2002) Dialectic in Marxism and critical realism. In Eds Brown, A, Fleetwood, S & Roberts, J: Critical Realism and Marxism. London: Routledge.

Collins, C, McCrory, M, Mackenzie, M & McCartney, G (2015) Social theory and health inequalities: Critical realism and a transformative activist stance. *Social Theory and Health* 13 377–396.

Commission on Social Determinants of Health (2008) Closing the Gap in a Generation. Geneva; World Health Organization.

Creaven, S (2007) Emergentist Marxism: Dialectical Philosophy and Social Theory. London; Routledge.

Crook, S, Paluski, J & Waters, M (1992) Postmodernization: Changes in Advanced Society. London; Sage.

Danemark, B, Ekstrom, M, Jacobsen, L & Karlsson, J (2002) Explaining Society: Critical Realism in the Social Sciences. London; Routledge.

Dawe, A (1970) The two sociologies. *British Journal of Sociology* 21 207–218.

Domhoff, G & Ballard, H (Eds) (1968) C Wright Mills and the Power Elite. Boston; Beacon Press.

Dorling, D (2013) Unequal Health: The Scandal of our Times. Bristol, UK; Policy Press.

Doyal, L & Doyal, L (1999) The British National Health Service: A tarnished moral vision. *Health Care Analysis* 7 263–276.

Dronkers, J & Schiff, H (2007) Elites. In Ed Ritzer, G: The Blackwell Encyclopedia of Sociology. Oxford; Blackwell.

Eagleton, T (2011) Why Marx was Right. New Haven, CT; Yale University Press.

Elias, N (1931/1996) The Germans: Power Struggles and the Development of Habitus in the Nineteenth and Twentieth Centuries. Cambridge, UK; Polity Press.

Engels, F (1999) The Conditions of the Working Class in England in 1844. Oxford; Oxford University Press.

Evans, G & Tilley, J (2017) The New Politics of Class: The Political Exclusion of the British Working Class. Oxford; Oxford University Press.

Eyler, J (1979) Victorian Social Medicine: The Ideas and Methods of William Farr. Baltimore, MD; Johns Hopkins University Press.

Featherstone, M (1991) In pursuit of the postmodern: an introduction. *Theory, Culture and Society* (specials issue on postmodernism) 5 2–3.

Fitzpatrick, R & Chandola, T (2000) Health. In Eds Halsey, A & Webb, J: Twentieth Century British Social Trends. London; Macmillan.

Fitzpatrick, R & Speed, E (2018) Variations in disease patterns in human society. In Ed Scambler, G: Sociology as Applied to Health and Medicine. London; Palgrave McMillan.

Fleetwood, S (2002) What kind of theory is Marx's theory of labour value? A critical realist enquiry. In Eds Brown, A, Fleetwood, S & Roberts, J: Critical Realism and Marxism. London; Routledge.

Foucault, M (1977) Language, Counter-Memory, Practice. Ithaca, NY; Cornell University Press.

Foucault, M (1980) Power/Knowledge. Brighton, UK; Harvester.

Foucault, M (1989) The Birth of the Clinic. London; Routledge.

Fox, N (2015) Personal health technologies, micropolitics and resistance: A new materialist analysis. *Health* 21(2) 136–153

Freidson, E (1970) Profession of Medicine. New York; Dodd, Mead & Co.

Galbraith, K (1992) The Culture of Contentment. London; Sinclair-Stevenson.

Garfinkel, H (1967) Studies in Ethnomethodology. Englewood Cliffs, NJ; Prentice-Hall.

Garthwaite, K (2016) Hunger Pains: Life Inside Foodbank Britain. Bristol, UK; Bristol University Press.

Gerhardt, U (1987) Ideas about Illness: An Intellectual and Political Theory of Medical Sociology. London; Macmillan.

Gerhardt, U (2002) Talcott Parsons: An Intellectual Biography. Cambridge, UK; Cambridge University Press.

Giddens, A (1990) Consequences of Modernity. Cambridge, UK; Polity Press.

Goffman, E (1968a) Asylums: Essays on the Social Situation of Mental Patients and Other Inmates. Harmondsworth, UK; Penguin.

Goffman, E (1968b) Stigma: the Management of Spoiled Identity. Harmondsworth, UK; Penguin.

Goffman, E (1969) The Presentation of Self in Everyday Life. Harmondsworth, UK; Penguin.

Goffman, E (1971) Relations in Public: Microstudies of the Social Order. New York; Basic Books.

Goldthorpe, J (2016) Sociology as a Population Science. Cambridge, UK; Cambridge University Press.

Gouldner, A (1970) The Coming Crisis of Western Sociology. New York; Equinox Books.

Habermas, J (1975) Legitimation Crisis. London; Heinemann.

Habermas, J (1981) New social movements. *Telos* 49 33–37.

Habermas, J (1984) Theory of Communicative Action, Volume 1: Reason and the Rationalization of Society. London; Heinemann.

Habermas, J (1987) Theory of Communicative Action, Volume 2: Lifeworld and System: A Critique of Functionalist Reason. Cambridge, UK; Polity Press.

Habermas, J (1989) The New Conservatism. Cambridge, UK; Polity Press.

Habermas, J (1994) The Past as Future. Cambridge, UK; Polity Press.

Henderson, L (1935) Physican and patient as a social system. *New England Journal of Medicine* 212 819–823.

Honneth, A (2017) The Idea of Socialism. Cambridge, UK; Polity Press.

Hopkins, A (1987) The causes and precipitation of seizures. In Ed Hopkins, A: Epilepsy. London; Chapman Hall.

Horkheimer, M & Adorno, T (1972) Dialectic of Enlightenment. New York; Herder & Herder.

Jessop, B (1998) Karl Marx. In Ed Stones, R: Key Sociological Thinkers. London; Macmillan.

Keat, R & Urry, J (1975) Social Theory and Science. London; Routledge & Kegan Paul.

Krieger, N (2017) Health equity and the fallacy of treating causes of population health as if they sum to 100%. *American Journal of Public Health* 107 541–549.

Landes, D (1998) Wealth and Poverty of Nations. London; Little, Brown & Co.

Lawson, T (1997) Economics and Reality. London; Routledge.

Lawson, T (2014) A speeding up of the rate of social change? Power, technology, resistance, globalisatoion and the good society. In Ed Archer, M: Late Modernity: Trajectories towards Morphogenetic Society. New York; Springer.

Leys, D & Player, S (2011) The Plot Against the NHS. London; The Merlin Press.

Link, B & Phelan, J (2001) Conceptualizing stigma. *Annual Review of Sociology* 27 363–385.

Lockwood, D (1964) System integration and social integration. In Eds Zollschan, G & Hirsch, W: Explorations in Social Change. London; Houghton Mifflin.

Lupton, D (2012) M-Health and health promotion: The digital cyborg and surveillance society. *Social Theory and Health* 10 229–244.

Lupton, D (2015) Digital Sociology. London; Routledge.

Lupton, D (2016) The Quantified Self: A Sociology of Self-Tracking. Cambridge, UK; Polity Press.

Lyotard, J-J (1984) The Postmodern Condition. Manchester; Manchester University Press.

Maldano-Torres, N (2007) On the coloniality of being: Contributions to the development of a concept. *Cultural Studies* 21 240–270.

Marmot, M (2004) Status Syndrome: How your Place on the Social Gradient Directly Affects your Health. London; Bloomsbury.

Marmot Review (2010) Fair Society, Healthy Lives: Strategic Review of Health Inequalities in England Post-2010. London; Department of Health.

Marx, K (1933) Wage Labour and Capital. London; Lawrence & Wishart.

Marx, K (1973) Grundrisse: Foundations of the Critique of Political Economy. Harmondsworth, UK; Penguin.

Mason, P (2015) Postcapitalism: A Guide to the Future. London; Allen Lane.

McDonnell, O (2013) Social constructionism. In Eds Gabe, J & Monaghan, L: Key Concepts in Medical Sociology. London; Sage.

McKeown, T (1979) The Role of Medicine: Dream, Mirage or Nemesis, 2nd ed. Oxford; Blackwell.

Mead, GH (1934) Mind, Self and Society: From the Standpoint of a Social Behaviourist. Chicago, IL; Chicago University Press.

Merton, T (1968) Social Theory and Social Structure. New York; Free Press.

Miliband, R (1961) Parliamentary Socialism. London; The Merlin Press.

Mills, CW (1956) The Power Elite. New York; Oxford University Press.

Mills, CW (1963) The Sociological Imagination. Harmondsworth, UK; Penguin.

Monbiot, G (2016) No country with a McDonalds can remain a democracy. *Guardian* 6 December.

Mortimer, I (2014) Centuries of Change. London; Bodley Head.

Navidi, S (2017) Superhubs: How the Financial Elite and their Networks Rule our World. St. Ives, UK; Nicholas Brealey Publishing.

Nettleton, S (2013) The Sociology of Health and Illness, 3rd ed. Cambridge, UK; Polity Press.

Nicolson, M & McLaughlin, C (1987) Social constructionism and medical sociology: A reply to M.R.Bury. *Sociology of Health and Illness* 9 107–126.

Nicolson, M & McLaughlin, C (1988) Social constructionism and medical sociology: A study of the vascular theory of multiple sclerosis. *Sociology of Health and Illness* 10 234–261.

Norrie, A (2010) Dialectic and Difference: Dialectical Critical Realism and the Grounds of Justice. London; Routledge.

Office for National Statistics (ONS) (2007) Trends in Life Expectancy by Social Class 1972–2005. London; Office for National Statistics.

Office of National Statistics (ONS) (2012) Intercensal Mortality Rates by NS-SEC, 2001–2010. London; Office for National Statistics.

Olafsdottir, S (2013) Social construction and health. In Ed Cockerham, W: Medical Sociology on the Move: New Directions in Theory. New York; Springer.

Oliver, M (1990) The Politics of Disablement. Basingstoke, UK; Macmillan.

Oxfam (2014) Working for the Few. London; Oxfam.

Pakulski, J & Waters, M (1996) The Death of Class. London; Sage.

Parsons, T (1937) The Structure of Social Action: A Study in Social Theory with Special Reference to a Group of Recent European Writers. New York; McGraw-Hill.

Parsons, T (1951) The Social System. London; Routledge.

Petersen, A (2012) Foucault, health and healthcare. In Ed Scambler, G: Contemporary Theorists for Medical Sociology. London; Routledge.

Picketty, T (2014) Capital in the Twenty-First Century. Cambridge, MA; Harvard University Press.

Pollock, A (2005) NHS Plc: The Privatisation of our Health Care. London; Verso.

Porpora, D (2015) Reconstructing Sociology: The Critical Realist Approach. Cambridge, UK; Cambridge University Press.

Preobrazhensky, E (1964) The New Economics. Oxford; Oxford University Press.

Ritzer, G (2001) The McDonaldisation of American sociology: A metasociological anaylsis. In Ritzer, G: Explorations in Social Theory: From Metatheorizing to Rationalization. London; Sage.

Ritzer, G (2003) Contemporary Sociological Theory and its Classical Roots. New York; McGraw-Hill.

Roberts, C & Cox, M (2003) Health and Disease in Britain: From Prehistory to the Present Day. Stroud, UK: Sutton Publishing Ltd.

Rorty, R (1989) Contingency, Irony and Solidarity. Cambridge, UK; Cambridge University Press.

Said, E (1995) Orientalism: Western Conceptions of the Orient. London; Penguin.

Sayer, A (2015) Why We Can't Afford the Rich. Bristol, UK; Policy Press.

Savage, M (2015) Social Class in the 21st Century. Birmingham, UK; Penguin.

Scambler, G (1987) Habermas and the power of medical expertise. In Ed Scambler, G: Sociological Theory and Medical Sociology. London; Tavistock.

Scambler, G (1989) Epilepsy. London; Tavistock.

Scambler, G (1996) The 'project of modernity' and the parameters for a critical sociology: An argument with illustrations from medical sociology. *Sociology* 30 567–581.

Scambler, G (2001a) Introduction: unfolding themes of an incomplete project. In Ed Scambler, G: Habermas, Critical Theory and Health. London; Routledge.

Scambler, G (2001b) Habermas, Critical Theory and Health. London; Routledge.

Scambler, G (2002) Health and Social Change. Buckingham, UK; Open University Press.

Scambler, G (2004) Re-framing stigma: Felt and enacted stigma and challenges to the sociology of chronic and disabling conditions. *Social Theory and Health* 2 29–46.

Scambler, G (2005a) Medical sociology: Past, present and future. In Ed Scambler, G: Medical Sociology. Major Themes in Health and Social Welfare, Volume One. London; Routledge.

Scambler, G (2005b) Sport and Society: History, Power and Culture. Maidenhead, UK; Open University Press.

Scambler, G (2006) Sociology, social structure and health-related stigma. *Psychology, Health and Medicine* 11 288–295.

Scambler, G (2009) Health-related stigma. *Sociology of Health and Illness* 31 441–455.

Scambler, G (2012a) Health inequalities. *Sociology of Health and Illness* 34 130–146.

Scambler, G (2012b) Archer, morphogenesis and the role of agency in the sociology of health inequalities. In Ed Scambler, G: Contemporary Theorists for Medical Sociology. London; Routledge.

Scambler, G (2012c) Resistance in unjust times: Archer, structured agency and the sociology of health inequalities. *Sociology* 47 1 142–156.

Scambler, G (2013) Archer and 'vulnerable fractured reflexivity': A neglected social determinant of health. *Social Theory and Health* 11(3) 302–315.

Scambler, G (2014) Medical sociology in the twenty-first century. *Contemporary Sociology* 43.

Scambler, G (2015) Jurgen Habermas: Health and healing across the lifeworld-system divide. In Ed Collyer, F: The Palgrave Handbook of Social Theory in Health, Illness and Medicine. London; Palgrave-Macmillan.

Scambler, G (In Press) Heaping blame on shame – stigma and deviance in neoliberal times. *The Sociological Review.*

Scambler, G, Afentouli, P & Selai, C (2010) Discerning biological, psychological and social mechanisms in the impact of epilepsy on the individual: A framework and exploration. In Eds Scambler, G & Scambler, S: New Directions in the Sociology of Chronic and Disabling Conditions: Assaults on the Lifeworld. London; Palgrave Macmillan.

Scambler, G & Goraya, A (1994) Movements for change: The new public health. *Critical Public Health* 5 4–10.

Scambler, G & Higgs, P (1999) Stratification, class and health: Class relations and health inequalities in high modernity. *Sociology* 32 275–291.

Scambler, G & Higgs, P (2001) The dog that didn't bark: Taking class seriously in the health inequalities debate. *Social Science and Medicine* 52 157–159.

Scambler, G & Kelleher, D (2006) New social and health movements: Issues of representation and change. *Critical Public Health* 16 219–231.

Scambler, G & Scambler, S (2013) Marx, critical realism and health inequalities. In Ed Cockerham, W: Medical Sociology on the Move: New Directions in Theory. New York; Springer.

Scambler, G & Scambler, S (2015) Theorizing health inequalities: The untapped potential of dialectical critical realism. *Social Theory and Health* 13 340–354.

Scambler, G, Scambler, S & Speed, E (2014) Civil society and the Health and Social Care Act in England and Wales: Theory and praxis for the twenty-first century. *Social Science and Medicine* 123 210–216.

Schutz, A (1962) Collected Papers Volume 1. The Hague; Martinus Nijhoff.

Schutz, A (1964) Collected Papers Volume 2. The Hague; Martinus Nijhoff.

Schutz, A (1970) Phenomenology of the Social World. Evanston, IL; Northwestern University Press.

Scott, J (1991) The Ruling Class. Cambridge, UK; Polity Press.

Scott, J (2008) Modes of power and the re-coneptualisation of elites. In Eds Savage, M & Williams, K: Remembering Elites. Oxford; Blackwell.

Scott-Samuel, A (2012) Where the NHS is heading. *Letter in Guardian*, 20 January.

Seeman, M (1959) On the meaning of alienation. *American Sociological Review* 24 783–791.

Seigrist, J (2009) Unfair exchange and health: Social bases of stress-related diseases. *Social Theory and Health* 7 305–317.

Sitton, J (1996) Recent Marxian Theory: Class Formation and Social Conflict in Contemporary Capitalism. New York; State University of New York Press.

Spivak, G (1990) Can the subaltern speak? In Eds Nelson, C & Grossberg, L: Marxism and the Interpretation of Culture. Chicago; University of Illinois Press.

Stalder, F (2006) Manual Castells: The Theory of the Network Society. Cambridge, UK; Polity Press.

Standing, G (2011) The Precariat: The New Dangerous Class. London; Bloomsbury.

Standing, G (2017) Basic Income and How We Can Make it Happen. Birmingham, UK; Penguin.

Streeck, W (2016) How Will Capitalism End? London; Verso.

Taylor, R & Rieger, A (1985) Medicine as a social science: Rudolf Virchow on the typhus epidemic in Upper Silesia. *International Journal of Health Services* 15 549–559

The Equality Trust (2016a) The scale of economic inequality in the UK. www.equalitytrust.org.uk/scale-economic-inequality-uk

The Equality Trust (2016b) How has inequality changed? www.equalitytrust.org.uk/how-has-inequality-changed

Therborn, G (2014) The Killing Fields of Inequality. Cambridge, UK; Polity Press.

Thomas, C (2007) Sociologies of Disability and Illness: Contested Ideas in Disability Studies and Medical Sociology. London; Palgrave-Macmillan.

Thompson, J (1995) The Media and Modernity: A Social Theory of the Media. Cambridge, UK; Polity Press.

Turner, B (1995) Medical Power and Social Knowledge, 2nd ed. London; Sage.

Tyler, I (2013) Revolting Subjects: Social Abjection and Resistance in Neoliberal Britain. London; Zed Books.

Tyler, I (Forthcoming) The Stigma Doctrine.

Urry, J (2016) What is the Future? Cambridge, UK; Polity Press.

Vygotsky, L (1934) Thought and Language. Cambridge, MA; MIT Press.

Weiland, W (1975) Diagnose. Berlin; de Gruyter.

Wilkinson, R & Pickett, K (2009) The Spirit Level: Why More Equal Societies Almost Always do Better. London; Allen Lane.

Williams, R (1977) Marxism and Literature. Oxford; Oxford University Press.

Williams, H (2006) Britain's Power Elites: The Rebirth of a Ruling Class. London; Constable.

Williams, S (2012) Health and medicine in the information age: Castells, informational capitalism and the network society. In Ed Scambler, G: Contemporary Theorists for Medical Sociology. London; Routledge.

Winlow, S, Hall, S, Treadwell, J & Briggs, D (2015) Riots and Political Protest: Notes from the Post=Political Present. London; Routledge.

Winlow, J, Hall, S & Treadwell, J (2017) The Rise of the Right: English Nationalism and the Transformation of Woprking-Class Politics. Bristol, UK; Policy Press.

Wittgenstein, L (1958) Philosophical Investigations, 2nd ed. Oxford; Blackwell.

Wynter, S (2003) Unsettling the coloniality of being/power/truth/freedom: After man, its overrepresentation – an argument. *CR: The New Centennial Review* 3 257–337.

Yuill, C (2005) Marx: Capitalism, alienation and health. *Social Theory and Health* 3 126–143.

Zizek, S (2016) Against the Double Blackmail. Milton Keynes, UK; Allen Lane.

Index